BELOW THE BELT

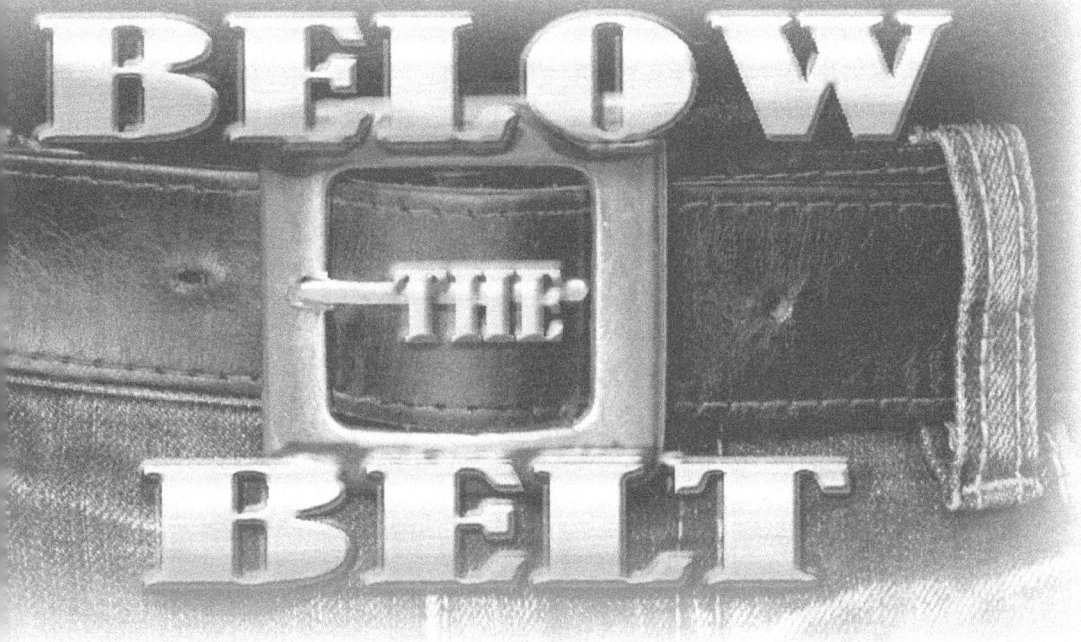

Experiences with Prostate Cancer

First published by Busybird Publishing 2015
Copyright © 2015 Busybird Publishing
ISBN 978-0-9925547-3-6

Chief Editors: Les Zigomanis, Marieclaire Baird
Poetry Editor: Krystle Herdy
Assistant Editors: Rebecca Courtney, Terri Giuretis, Ariel Skippen, Courtney Baxter, Erin Dite, Shevon Higgins, Klara Cole, Johanna Boutros.
Proofreader: Tom O'Connell, Blaise van Hecke

Cover image: Kev Howlett, Busybird Publishing
Cover design: Kev Howlett, Busybird Publishing
Layout and typesetting: Busybird Publishing

Busybird Publishing
2/118 Para Road
Montmoency, Victoria
Australia 3094
www.busybird.com.au

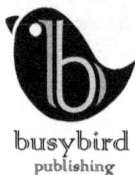

DISCLAIMER: The producers of this book, and the authors of the stories are not medical professionals. It is not intended as a medical diagnostic tool, but rather a guide to help anyone facing prostate cancer. Always seek medical advice and second opinions where your health is concerned.

Contents

Foreword:
The Importance of Support

Peter Gebert

Men in Australia with prostate cancer are being deprived of a well-structured and supportive network of support groups.

Support groups are a proven resource, providing men who have prostate cancer and their families with valuable information and firsthand experience about the journey they are on or are about to commence. Yet, too few men know that support groups exist, or the important role a support group can play.

It is estimated that in 2012, over 20,000 Australian men were diagnosed with prostate cancer. Of this number, a little more than 1,000 Australian men availed themselves to the services of the 159 support groups in Australia.

It is startling to think that 95% of the newly diagnosed men in Australia miss out on a valuable, free service that might make a real difference in their lives. More than 8,000 Australians believe there is value because they either still attend or receive regular information about the latest matters around prostate cancer.

So, what does a support group offer and what can one expect when attending a support group meeting?

The current 159 Prostate Cancer Foundation of Australia-affiliated support groups are all run by volunteers, the majority being men and their partners who are still living the Prostate

Cancer journey. These individuals give their time and experience so that others may have better outcomes if they are touched by this all-too-common disease.

Most of these groups meet monthly, either at night or during the day, and details can be found at www.pcfa.org.au.

Research from Canada suggests that men who attend Prostate Cancer Support Groups cope better with their medical situation. This is because they are better informed and educated about the various issues that being diagnosed and treated for prostate cancer can bring on and what medical terms mean when they are raised by the various medical professionals during their journey.

This is very valuable when a man and his partner are about to make a life-changing decision. It involves nothing more than talking to, listening to, and asking questions of other men who are still living after undertaking various forms of disease management or treatment currently available in Australia. Who better to talk to if you are about to embark on a trip than someone who has been there and back?

Support groups in Australia are well-structured with men and women volunteers who not only run the groups, but grow and support them in their state, and on a national level try to bring consistency and process and ensure their groups are up to date with all the latest information provided by the PCFA, Cancer Councils, Andrology Australia and Beyond Blue, to name a few.

Men and their partners are starting to become more engaged around helping themselves and even more are trying to get the word to other men in their communities about the value of early detection and appropriate treatment.

The wider use of the internet allows more and more people to source information (both good and bad), but it is spreading the word that there are more men just like them out there living with prostate cancer. The other good thing is that men can now make an informed choice on what they want to do rather than just accept what they are told and live with the outcomes for their remaining days, no matter how long. Many men also find a lot of benefit in talking about the side effects they may have from various treatments with others who are still living with them or have overcome them.

Ages of men at support groups vary from mid-40s to 80s, so there is usually someone that will relate to your situation. The sizes of groups vary from 5 to 80 with the average size in Victoria being 13 attendees.

Most people attend groups both to learn about cancer and its treatments, and to deal with the emotional, social, practical and personal effects of having the disease. They may be looking for information, encouragement, inspiration, hope for survival, or ideas about how to get the best outcome and maintain their quality of life. Some people don't want to attend meetings at all but it is important for them to realise that the 'support group' is a network they can connect with and talk to like-minded people by phone and receive relevant information via newsletters etc.

Recent research funded by The Cancer Council has found that the top reasons why people join a support group are to:

- know they aren't alone
- hear about current medical research
- become more informed about cancer treatment and side effects
- compare their experiences and learn how other people deal with cancer, and
- relax with others who can empathise with what they're going through.

Many groups also spend considerable time running awareness events in their community, promoting awareness of prostate cancer and the resources offered by the individual support group.

For example, in the Diamond Valley in Melbourne the local group has held the following events over the years:

- Golf days
- Art exhibitions
- Music concerts
- Sunday walks
- Health awareness evenings at local YMCAs.

This group has won local community awards for its work and had various members of the group win local and national awards for their services to prostate cancer and their community.

The Diamond Valley Prostate Cancer Support Group meets every third Monday of the month at the Montmorency RSL at 7.00 pm. All visitors are welcome.

Peter Gebert
– Support Group Convenor.

Active Surveillance

David Howell

My father died of prostate and bladder cancer. It was a horrific and heart-wrenching experience watching him in his last days. He'd always been a very strong, active man and now the ravages of age and cancer had reduced him to a man now totally dependent on the care of the palliative nurses. The dichotomy of these images still resides in my memory. So when a couple of acquaintances were diagnosed with cancer – one with prostate cancer and the other with bladder cancer – I thought I should get a check-up to see how my prostate was going.

My regular GP is female and I didn't know whether she'd perform a digital rectal examination of my prostate. The thought of a female doctor checking my prostate was not the concern – I was more worried it would cause *her* embarrassment. I asked if she did the digital examinations and explained that if she didn't I understood and would instead see one of her male colleagues at the surgery. She said it wasn't a problem for her at all and she was glad I'd decided to have a check-up.

After the examination, she informed me that she had detected an abnormality, a roughened area on the left side of my prostate gland, and that she would like me to see a specialist for further tests. I knew of an excellent urologist already through an acquaintance, so I was referred to him.

My heart was beating fast by the time I got home and telephoned the urologist's rooms to make an appointment. Luckily, I only had a fortnight to wait before I saw him. During that time, I checked medical texts and reliable medical sources on the internet to find out more about prostate cancer. I knew a little about prostate cancer but not a great deal about the specifics, such as how it is actually diagnosed, apart from a digital examination and the blood tests. The journal articles I read talked about different studies and treatment outcomes, as well as the side effects of some treatments. I heard a radio interview where a specialist was discussing prostate cancer treatments and worldwide studies; he stressed the need to have an experienced surgeon. Like most surgery, the more experienced the surgeon, either in manual or robotic surgery techniques, the better. The number of successful operations increases the skill level and the odds of a more positive outcome, and hopefully reduces the potential side effects such as urinary incontinence and impotence, although there is also a degree of luck in any surgical procedure. It was scary knowing that I might have cancer; it brought back memories of my dad and his suffering.

Parking the car and walking into the urologist's building was a normal 'visit the doctor' type experience. After I'd filled in the new-patient information form, I joined the large group of men – some with their wives – in the waiting room. It was so quiet, I thought I should say something to someone because the silence was unsettling. I wished I'd brought my wife along, just so I wasn't alone. One lady tried to engage her partner in a conversation about an article in the magazine she was reading, no doubt to take his mind off his appointment.

Everyone was there for probably the same reason, some pale looking, others unruffled, some were in and out of the various specialists' rooms quickly, while others took longer.

Most were much older than me. I looked at these men and thought, *What an interesting mix.* Outside, we'd probably not cross paths, yet here at the urologists' it didn't matter who you were. Prostate cancer was a real equaliser.

Eventually, the specialist called my name. He was a tall, pleasant-looking young man. He shook my hand, introduced himself, then asked me to follow him. This simple introduction immediately reduced my anxiety a little. He had the personal touch. I liked that. It mattered in this situation.

After the preliminaries, he wanted to know what had prompted me to have my GP perform a digital examination of my prostate, as I was a 'relatively young man'. I was not having pain or any trouble passing urine or erectile problems, but I did have a family history. He understood my reasoning, especially after my acquaintances' experiences, and then proceeded to examine me. I must admit that my GP's digital examination was much less painful and probing than his!

We sat down and he explained that his examination concurred with my GP's diagnosis. He'd found my prostate gland to be of normal size, with the roughened abnormality to be slightly larger than what she'd found. He let that sink in and then said that I needed a blood test to check the PSA levels in my blood. PSA is a protein normally released by the prostate. Blood tests measure the levels of this protein, but they are not definitive of whether a man has prostate cancer or not. The blood test just provides a further set of data to assist in identifying if cancer is present. He then told me that biopsies (the use of very fine needles to remove very small pieces of prostate gland tissue for microscopic examination) were also required for definitive diagnosis.

He talked about various treatment modalities, but I'd already made my mind up to ask for surgery if he discovered I had prostate cancer, although I didn't say so at this stage.

After paying my account, I checked the pathology request form and found a location nearby; not wanting to delay the process, I headed straight there. Yes, they're nearly always busy, but I was in luck, as there were only two people waiting. Blood sample taken, I headed home.

I called my wife and informed her of the findings and that I'd already had the blood test. Both of us talked positively, knowing that I couldn't possibly have cancer! Then I went to university; I was doing an Honours Degree in Environmental Science, and life went on. I kept everything to myself; I would be all right. I was pretty tough. I was bulletproof.

My wife wanted to come with me to my next appointment with the urologist, but I felt I'd be a man and handle it all myself. This caused friction. My wife just wanted to be there for me and I was closing her out. As the appointment drew nearer, I got more fidgety and worried about what I might hear; I relented and asked her to accompany me.

My urologist greeted me the same as he had before and introduced himself to my wife. He was pleased that I had brought her and told us my PSA reading was high but not seriously so. He stressed that a needle biopsy was the next part of the diagnosis, because PSA levels can vary for a number of reasons. Tissue samples might pick up cancer cells if they were present, thereby confirming the diagnosis.

I felt worried he was preparing me for the possibility of the statement, 'You have prostate cancer.' But I had every faith in him; he was professional and I liked him. I told him from the outset that I would be guided by his opinion and experience.

Before I'd left his rooms, an appointment had been made for my prostate biopsy and I was given a prescription for antibiotics. He had already fully explained that the procedure required me to have a minor general anesthetic and up to 12 biopsy needles would be inserted into my prostate via a probe in my rectum. I had to start a course of very strong antibiotics prior to the procedure to eliminate the possibility of an infection from the needles passing through my bowel wall.

I arrived for my biopsy a week later and noted a number of older gentlemen attired like me, in the requisite white 'open at the back' gown and terry-towelling dressing gown, some with partners, some toughing it out alone, all waiting for similar procedures. I am not sure if the cold chill was from the atmosphere of the sterile waiting room or simply from the open-backed gown!

I had an intravenous cannula inserted by the anaesthetist – a nice man for the short period I saw him, because within about thirty seconds I knew nothing more.

I woke in recovery and gradually regained my composure. My darling wife then drove me home. I cannot say that I was sore after the biopsy, although I had a feeling like a deep cramp in my lower abdomen for a couple of days – not painful but like a muscle strain. I'd read all the literature about abstaining from sex for a period of time (a week?) and that there might be blood in any ejaculation – they weren't wrong. It is an extremely sickening feeling to see dark brown-coloured ejaculate. I freely admit I nearly passed out when I saw it. 'There might be blood' doesn't really prepare you for the situation. It cleared over a few days.

Then it was back to my specialist. My wife accompanied me. He explained that a couple of the needles had picked up some cancer cells; these had been identified as a slow-growing, less aggressive type. The results were conclusive – I did have prostate cancer.

This hit me! The 'C' word – I'd kind of known somehow that the needle biopsy would show I had cancer, although I'd still hoped otherwise. My body and mind were numb. The doctor had seen this reaction many times before and waited. My wife was upset but controlled herself, being strong for me.

'Just cut it out, remove my prostate,' was my ham-fisted immediate response to the news. I'd previously decided that having surgery was the definitive treatment, thinking that if it was out, it couldn't hurt you!

The urologist reiterated that I was a 'young man' and that there were many alternatives to surgery, as there were complications associated with all the treatment options.

He went on to explain all the treatments and any issues associated with them. Radical prostatectomy, the surgical removal of the prostate gland by 'open surgery' or a 'keyhole' robotic procedure;

radiation therapy, involving a lengthy period of time – weeks of going into Peter Mac for beams of x-rays to be fired into the prostate gland; brachytherapy, where rice grain-sized radioactive seeds are placed in the prostate gland or needles containing radioactive matter which are inserted into the prostate for a period of time; high-focused ultrasound (HIFU) or hormonal and chemotherapy. 'Watchful Waiting' and 'Active Surveillance' were two other options he talked about.

Because of my age and the fact that my cancer was of the less aggressive type, he wanted me to consider all the treatment options before making an informed decision. He arranged for me to visit the Peter MacCallum Cancer Centre and talk with an oncologist so that I was completely informed. He also gave me a booklet so that I could read about prostate cancer, the treatments, and all the terminology.

Going to Peter Mac was a daunting experience. Just knowing it was the 'cancer hospital' was confronting. I had to fill out a 'new patient' form, I was given a Peter Mac patient appointment wallet, and then I had to find where I needed to go for my appointment with the oncologist.

Once again, I was blessed, as he was also an extremely lovely, caring man. He reiterated what I had already been told about radiation and chemotherapy, gladly answered my questions, and also provided me with a different booklet on prostate cancer. Before leaving, he stressed that I could contact him if I had any further questions, as he understood that I had to make a decision on which way to proceed. He gave me all the facts so that I could make an informed decision on what to do.

My next urology appointment was decision time. Although I still thought about surgery, I felt I understood all the pros and cons now, the 'what ifs' around all the treatment modalities. I had decided to make my final decision after talking to my urologist. Once again, he walked me through all the treatments, talked about the blood test and biopsy results and my cancer's expected progression. Because my cancer was a slow-growing one, and following discussions with the urologist, the oncologist and my family and my readings of the extensive booklets the doctors had provided, I chose to go into the 'Active Surveillance' category, which involved ongoing blood tests, needle biopsies, and regular visits to the urologist. I also consented to having my progress recorded on a database so that any information gained might assist with the treatment of prostate cancer in other men.

After the initial shock of being told I had cancer and coming to terms with that, life was pretty much back to normal. I finished my Honours Degree and worked at various paid and volunteer jobs. I always became apprehensive around the time of the next blood test or biopsy. It was difficult not to get stressed, wondering what each test would find.

I had a new type of needle biopsy called a 'Trans-perineal' biopsy, which goes through the perineum, the area between the scrotum and the anus. This biopsy looked at my prostate from a different direction and it discovered that my prostate now had two types of cancer – a slow-growing cancer and a highly aggressive form. A new treatment strategy was required.

My wife and I met the urologist in July 2012 to discuss the results, and, consequently, I made the decision to have radical robotic surgery after my urologist clearly explained what the surgery entailed. It is 'keyhole' surgery, where five small holes are made and the procedure is done through these. It also normally meant a shorter time in hospital and fewer complications, such as pain and bleeding or time off work. We also discussed my weight, as I had quite a layer of fat around my abdomen, and I agreed to lose weight before the operation.

The urologist then arranged for me to meet with his nursing team and a physiotherapist in mid-August. The nurse's task was to explain all the issues around urinary catheters and incontinence, my hospital stay and afterwards, how I was to manage with the urinary catheter at home, and the incontinence pads that I would need to wear after the catheter's removal. She told me that there were a number of pads on the market, but based on the experiences of their patients one brand was best. She showed me what the packet looked like and wrote down the name and the type of pad for men I would require.

The nurse went on to explain that, post-operatively, sex would be difficult, as erections are not possible, but that men can still have orgasms. This was news to me, as I thought men needed an erection to orgasm. She also explained how I wouldn't ejaculate when I had an orgasm or I might ejaculate a very small quantity of urine. This occurred because of the removal of the prostate and seminal vesicles and, I guess, the rearrangement of the 'plumbing'. She explained that erections do return over time and that the urologist would explain this further.

At the physiotherapy appointments, I was instructed how to find my pelvic floor muscles; this again involved a Digital Rectal Examination. I was unaware of this until the physiotherapist asked if she could do one. She needed to check the existing state of my pelvic floor muscles. My muscles were very strong according to her. I was then given exercises to prepare me for pre/post surgery, and I also had to keep a fluid balance chart so that my normal fluid intake and urine output was recorded. Before my surgery, I dieted and exercised, losing about 20kgs in four months, to make the surgery easier for both my urologist and myself.

On Friday, 16 November 2012, I arrived at the hospital for my operation and was home by Sunday morning. My surgery went really well. I woke with a urinary catheter bag and a surgical drainage bag in situ and the initial discomfort quickly eased. When the drainage bag was removed, I had a little discomfort, as the tube was drawn out from my abdomen. Then I was allowed to shower. This was a complicated affair, trying to manage the urinary catheter bag and shower, then having to change the bag and elastic straps, but I managed. Over time, I improved at this procedure. I had to have the catheter in and wear the collection bag for two weeks post-operatively to allow my bladder to heal.

Arriving home with the catheter bag strapped to my leg was uncomfortable. I felt like everyone could see it, but I quickly got used to wearing it and developed a routine around emptying it and changing over the bag when required, although I never got used to the smell of the bag and its attachments. Others couldn't smell it – I'd checked. It wasn't a urine smell but a sickly smell of the silicone catheter, the plastic urine bag, or the elastic straps holding the bag to my leg. I really looked forward to its removal. They were a long two weeks. I now have a very deep respect for anyone who has a catheter, especially those individuals who have them in long-term.

Prior to seeing my urologist post-operatively, I had an MRI to check that my surgery had completely healed. My urologist was pleased how the operation had progressed; unfortunately, the MRI had shown that there was still a small area at the mouth of my bladder that hadn't healed fully, so I had to keep wearing the urinary catheter for a further week. Blast! That was probably one of the hardest things; I just wanted to be free of it and its smell. I willed that next week away!

A week later, I met my urologist's nurse and she removed my urinary catheter. What a relief! Apart from the slight discomfort in withdrawing the tubing, it was gone. No more bag! I couldn't stop smiling. She acknowledged my pleasure and asked if I'd brought any incontinence pads. I started wearing them and, luckily, I only had to wear them for about eight weeks.

I saw my urologist and he was extremely happy with how I was progressing. I remarked to him how wonderful and at ease his nurse had made me feel both before and after the operation. I said I felt completely comfortable talking to her and that she was a credit to his practice.

I had my radical robotic prostatectomy over two years ago and have had no issues post-operatively. I returned to work seven weeks after my surgery. I remarked to my urologist that my orgasms are now even better than before the surgery, being more intense and longer lasting, and that I don't ejaculate. I continue to have blood tests six-monthly, and will eventually move to twelve-monthly, but my PSA readings have all been zero. At my last visit, in December 2013, my urologist said that I didn't need to see him again. This hit me, because I felt like I was losing a friend – he was such a nice guy.

I am extremely lucky to have a supportive wife and family, and to have had a wonderful team working with me throughout my cancer saga. We need the help of experts, and I am really pleased that my GP started me on the path to treatment and recovery.

It is important that men put aside their apathy, fear, or hubris and actually talk to their GP about prostate cancer and get to understand all the issues around it. This is an assassin waiting silently to strike, usually when we are older and less able to defend ourselves.

If I hadn't had that routine check with my GP in the first place, despite having no symptoms at all, I might not have had the life ahead of me that I do now.

Skinny Legs Pumping a Wild Bicycle

Debi Hamilton

i.   Once upon a time,
not so very long ago
and not far from here,
the wandering thread of one
man's life curled itself, without
thought, around a job,
a family, a bank account,
a car, a partner;
around a far-flung future;
around a body that was
careless, bullet-proof.

ii.   The thread had begun
more than fifty years before,
in the simple way
lives do, a new boy slipping
into the world to take up
the art of being
himself, finding his place in
a family, to
shape and be shaped by parents,
three brothers, and the business
of a river town.

iii.   Quite invisible
to itself, the thread unfurled
around camp fires
and lazy fishing trips; it
spooled from skinny legs pumping
a wild bicycle;
it looped reluctantly to
school, where it did its
homework and found itself drawn
to the family business.
It found its first love.

iv.   And so the boy grew
into a man, carrying
whatever this meant
into his boundless future.
He pulled the thread of his life
through a diploma,
then stretched it across the world
for two years. Later,
without learning the words for
the doings of his heart, he
married, had children.

v.   Years on, he would see
the cost of living without
reflection, but for
now the thread of his life ran
straight through the valley of hard
work, bigger houses,
business success. The sun shone
on his endeavours.
What went on inside himself
stayed in the realm of darkness,
alien to words.

vi.   Then one day the thread
snagged, stopped in its tracks
for a while. That world
he'd skated on proved to be
thin ice. His marriage ended—
a cold hard lesson.
He moved, he grew, he unearthed
some of the darkness.
The snagged thread disentangled,
found a new path to travel,
fell in love again.

vii.   Eleven years on,
        here is the scene in which the
        thread comes unravelled.
        Picture this—packing boxes
        stacked, Christmas carols on the
        radio; a new
        city, house, job are waiting.
        They are to marry.
        The phone rings. He has cancer.
        There's someone standing at the
        window with a scythe.

viii.   It seems a nightmare,
        like Christmas among the doomed.
        Deep in his body
        a vicious mystery has
        taken over. Surgery
        is booked and cancelled.
        His neck pain isn't tension.
        It is in his bones.
        They move house; find themselves on
        a new planet. He tries to
        write letters of hope.

ix.   The letters do help.
The doctors wheel in their guns—
oral castration
and a fierce battle plan.
The thread of his life seems frail,
then sturdy, then frail
again. He takes up talking,
starts meditating.
He has no time for whingers,
so whose are those tears he
sees in the mirror?

x.   Across town, the thread
of another life waits to
meet his. He has made
an appointment. She wonders
what he will bring, how she will
help. This is her work.
He comes in with his cape on—
the cape of coping.
Kind of Superman, she thinks.
She sees he is not ready
yet to take it off.

xi.   He doesn't take it
off, but he fiddles with it.
He is still working,
doing laps of the cosmos,
constructing all the castles
he wants to live in
forever with his sweetheart.
The castles become
urgent. He will build them with
the sheer force of his desire
to go on living.

xii.   He visits again.
The doctors' guns aren't working
but they have reserves.
Next stop, chemotherapy.
This time, they talk about the
cape, but he still can't
take it off. He's always worn
it; people admire
him in it. She says she'd like
him to leave it at the door
when he visits her.

xiii.   The next few months are
         conducted off-stage. He calls—
         his blood tests are clear.
         Weeks later, his sweetheart calls.
         He's disappeared. It's frightening.
         The woman rings him.
         He's not answering his phone.
         Afterwards she learns
         he'd taken off the cape, had
         to be treated for extreme
         identity loss.

xiv.   She rings him again.
         He's out of hospital; he's
         on the road to a
         ten-day retreat. They've called the
         artillery—he's having
         radiation, and
         is now on his way to find
         what the peace movement
         can offer as a back-up.
         In the face of all this, he's
         married his sweetheart.

xv.   Six months later, he's
back. The war for his body
goes on. He's weary.
His memory is dicey.
And as for sex—it's vanished.
Just like menopause,
she thinks. She's pleased to see he's
taken off the cape.
What does he need? A place to
cry, he says. His eyes leak tears.
They float in the room.

xvi.   How is he doing?
Strangely well. The war has knocked
down the wall between
him and the grace of the world.
Here's what matters—his sweetheart,
his children, all those
lives that thread themselves through his.
Would he go back, she
asks? No, in spite of it all.
And now there is Zytiga.
He is full of light.

Snakes and Ladders

Gaytana Adorna

You're wrenched from the known and hurled into a vortex of relentless appointments, tests and procedures.

There's so much to take in: complex information about staging, treatment options, possible outcomes, side effects, complications plus ... no guarantees. No assurances that once it's all done, that you'll be right again – free of prostate cancer; free to pick up where you left off and get on with enjoying your life.

When my husband's GP suggested he see a urologist as his PSA score had risen and was trending upwards, I thought, *Good. She's cautious.* It was such a low score, he was well – working at a demanding IT job, playing golf regularly – and had no symptoms, although very often, early prostate cancer has no symptoms. But I'm not a panic merchant.

After the first consultation David returned somewhat relieved. 'Small chance of cancer,' was his urologist's verdict after reviewing the case and examining David. But, to be on the safe side, he offered a biopsy, which David accepted. Now I was relieved. And confident. We awaited the results – David edgy but trying to hide his concerns. At one stage he did blurt out that he was sure it was cancer but I was still confident and hopeful of a less sinister outcome. Then, the results: cancer in each quadrant and a fairly aggressive cancer according to the Gleason score.

Five months earlier we'd celebrated my birthday and toasted life with a glass of bubbly to mark the end of chemotherapy after my breast cancer surgery. David admitted that there was a time when he'd thought I might not see another birthday. I'd had no idea he'd felt like that. But now he was smiling and confident. My dark hair was returning and I felt well. My oncologist still said we were on 'track for a cure'. Smiles all round. Dodged that one nicely. Now we were in the vortex again. Roles reversed.

I was dazed when prostate cancer was confirmed. All I could do was put my arms around David and say, 'I'm so sorry you have to go through this.' At least having supported me through surgery and chemo, he'd seen that cancer didn't have to be a death sentence and that the treatments are doable. I'd kept my sense of humour and we'd laughed a lot. David had been kind and comforting – kissing my bald head, saying, 'You're beautiful'. Now it was my turn to be there for him.

David decided on surgery – *thank God for a sensible decision* – as he was only in his fifties and wanted to give himself the best chance of a cure. I'd feared that he would be put off by the possibility of impotence or incontinence. The twin dreads that some experts love to trumpet, along with the fearful possibility of unnecessary cancer diagnoses and treatments, when 'most men die with, not of prostate cancer'. Men in their seventies or older maybe, not men in their fifties. And these well-meaning critics of the PSA test trot out the statistics. But David's not a statistic, he's a man with a lot more life he wants to live and interests and passions to pursue and travel to do; and he's my husband.

David knew the possible negatives of treatment; was given all the information, statistics, possible ways to deal with such problems and he felt that removing the cancer – hopefully before it spread – was the best option. I did too.

'I just want you alive,' I said.

I drove David to hospital then did housework to occupy myself and try to keep my eyes off the clock, as I waited for his urologist's call at the end of the surgery. He was prompt and had good news. Even better were the pathology results, a few days later: the cancer was contained and had not breached the capsule around the prostate. The lymph nodes were clear. *A great chance of cure. Joy!*

I raced to see David as he emerged from his anaesthetic, mumbling, 'Pain'.

'He's in pain,' I protested.

His urologist calmly made adjustments to the medications as he explained what he was administering. *Good man.*

A week later, when I brought David home, he still had the catheter in (these days they usually remove it before you leave hospital) and so we had to contend with the big overnight bag for the catheter and the more discreet one during the day; plus that first night, the question: do we swap the bags before he gets into his pyjamas or not and which leg first? Stumped, we fell about laughing and then got organised. Laughter and cuddles are a great help. Then, of course when they removed the catheter he was utterly incontinent for a while. But he did his pelvic floor exercises and gradually, fully recovered.

No incontinence, no impotence. No complications.

Then, the regular follow-up PSA tests and the tense wait, hoping he's still clear. A long-time friend of ours was diagnosed with prostate cancer a few months before David, and knowing my penchant for being well informed, he gave us his research folder to read. David declined the offer, preferring to talk with his specialist. So, I learned something David didn't. In some men, despite an early diagnosis before the cancer has spread, there is a genetic problem which seems to signal a poor prognosis. As nothing could then be done about the problem, I saw no reason to tell David of this. Waiting for the PSA test results worried him enough. He didn't need a vague, nasty possibility increasing the burden.

We don't keep secrets from each other. We're honest. Now I had a secret to keep.

Then, the milestones: one year – okay; three years, and his urologist was positive. Five years post cancer – that's a significant one. So often it's the five-year survival rate that's quoted to patients and media. *As if that's enough!* But five years and he was still clear. At ten years, his urologist, though conservative, suggested that David, need no longer see him. All indications were good. He said it wouldn't matter if David never had another PSA test, but it wouldn't hurt to have one occasionally. I told my secret.

It's 11 years now since treatment. David's well and even more active. He joined a bushwalking group and regularly walks many kilometres. Plus, having moved two years ago, we're creating a garden by hand from hard clay. And loving it. We celebrate the garden's increasing lushness and the birds that come regularly, feasting and now bringing their young; and the other visitors: the busy bees relishing all our flowering perennials, the butterflies and dragonflies. How lovely; how lucky we are.

We're neither smug, nor complacent; we're just grateful that we got another go at life. A number of friends were diagnosed around the same time as David. They too were younger men: in their fifties or barely sixty and glad their prostate cancer was found early. Sadly, not everyone gets a happy ending. Two of my girlfriends lost their husbands to prostate cancer. Every time the media erupts with an 'expert' criticising the PSA test, emphasising its limitations, and basically discouraging men from having the test, David gets furious. We both do. Men may die needlessly. David even emailed one health expert with his objections but got the standard reply. Now he just doesn't want to know about their views. He's still here because his GP believed in the test and her vigilance saved his life. He was lucky. Otherwise, he might have continued symptomless and unaware until it had spread and then his choices would have been limited, treatments would have only prolonged his life instead of cured him, he would have had unpleasant side effects and he would have then been in the medical vortex until he entered palliative care.

Despite their statistics and arguments, David's a believer. So am I. My community service announcement – encouraging men to have a PSA test and to ensure that they and their partners are fully informed – plays regularly on the community radio station I'm a member of and on which I prepare and present a weekly health and wellbeing programme.

We'd like all men to 'get lucky' and live.

Fear, Hope, Survival

John Dowsett

The worst day of my family life was the loss of a child in the birthing process. The worst day of *my* life was to be told that I had advanced prostate cancer and that the prognosis was that, without intervention, I would probably die in three to five years.

It started when I turned 60. I changed from a bi-annual to an annual check-up. In 1995, when I was 64, I went to my GP for my check-up and, after all the usual tests (he took my blood sample for blood counts, organ functions, etc.), he asked if I had ever had a PSA test because at my age it could be a good idea. I replied that I had not had one – what was it for? He explained that it was to check on the prostate gland's function so I agreed. Four days later, he contacted me to say that he had just seen the results. As he was leaving in a short time to go to Melbourne, he apologised for telling me over the phone but I had a very high reading and he had made an appointment for me with a urologist to examine the situation further.

This was the beginning of my cancer journey. I felt I was no longer in charge of my life and that the cancer was going to determine all my tomorrows. Fear and threat of death seemed to be the future. The urologist did all the primary examinations, which I didn't understand, a digital examination, another blood test and a further appointment. It wasn't until the next visit that I started wondering what was going on. The urologist told me that the prostate was enlarged and hard to the touch, the PSA reading was 96 and that I had prostate cancer. He informed me that it was a slow-growing cancer and that I had probably had it for more than a decade and to confirm these theories he wanted to do a biopsy and a bone scan.

The bone scan revealed that the cancer had spread to the bones and I was told that I had only two options: the first was to have hormone therapy consisting of Androcur tablets to be taken three times a day and Zoladex implants, one every four weeks; or the second was to have a sub-capsular orchidectomy, which is a form of castration. These treatments are a medical or a surgical treatment to stop the body's production of testosterone that feeds the cancer.

For a while, I avoided doing anything as I was in denial about death and wanted to just get on with living! The idea of tablets and implants was not my idea of a quality life and, as the results of both treatments would be the same, I opted for the orchidectomy, which I had in March 1996. It was uncertain how long starving the cancer would work through this treatment but I believed this option might give me a better quality of life. I also wondered how long I would have to live.

In April 1997, I joined a prostate cancer support group which had started in November 1995 and was run by the Cancer Council of Tasmania. I trained as a support person and later as a Cancer Connect Contact to talk with people on the telephone about their cancer. In 2001, I became the co-facilitator of the group and later facilitator until 2009, with a short break in 2008. In 2010, I started a group on the eastern shore of Hobart and resigned from that position in October 2011.

I strongly suggest that men of 40 years of age with a family history of prostate cancer, or men aged 50 and above should consult their GP about prostate cancer as an early diagnosis is best. I also recommend that, if diagnosed, joining a support group can be very helpful as you will hear the stories of other men and usually at least one man will have had similar experiences. Newcomers are given hope for their future. You will also hear of cases which are, in some ways, worse than your own, and find that nearly everyone in the group has time to support and bond with each other, no matter his own condition.

I started without any knowledge of this disease and full of fear. But, after being told we were only stalling the cancer, I have since survived over eighteen years. So, for me, diagnosis and treatment has led to an extended life – not cured, but the cancer held in check and under 'active surveillance' which, at age nearly 84, will probably be for the rest of my life.

Life's Path

Ron Turner

Death approaches
Like a threatening storm
In waves
Killing body tissues
Easing
Enough to give fresh hope
Only to return with greater force
And lay us low

We take for granted
Life
Until
The storm arrives
Deepening
Our depths of despair
As we traverse
The darkened trail of pity

In retrospect
Our minds compare
On life
Full of life
A boy
Fun-loving and mischievous
Remembering dare-devil deeds
Reflecting thoughts

Progressing to work
Looking towards change
Frustration
Through the years of toil
Visualising
The conquered quest
Our memories pale to recall
Those times

Forgotten are the times of worry
The non-events
What of deeds undone
Too late for many
Should I strive to amend
Those unjust deeds
Can I ever be forgiven
For this wasted life

What About Me?

Ross Henderson

When I turned 45, I felt I had reached a significant milestone in my life called 'middle age'. I was well in myself, single, free, with a good job, had a great family, marvellous friends, and was gay. I had 'come out' when I was 37 – late in life, for a whole variety of reasons – and was now enjoying my newly found freedom as a sexual man. I was finally integrated in a holistic sense.

I worked as a lecturer in the field of Counselling Psychology as a sole trader, consulting mostly to the government and not for profit sectors but also had some solid links to some large corporate organisations. I made enough money to live well. I loved dining out – one of my very favourite pastimes. I enjoyed the theatre, film, time away with friends and catching up with my family. Mum and Dad were well, my sister and her husband had three beautiful girls – my nieces, who just meant the world to me – and my younger brother and his wife were planning to start their own family.

One thing I did need to do something about was my fitness. Living by the sea I am constantly reminded of the beauty that comes with physical fitness, appreciating the bronzed, toned and well-sculpted bodies that parade my local area. Psychologically, things had been a little more problematic; I had experienced both troublesome anxiety and depression at a number of points in my life.

At 46 years of age, I decided to have that check-up that I had been postponing for the last 12 months. My GP is a gay man in his

60s, with a great sense of humour, skilled and knowledgeable, very caring, careful and wise, and he always took time to understand me. I love him; he is a marvellous man and a brilliant doctor.

Cholesterol, STIs, HIV status, blood pressure, blood sugars were all tested. My GP had also been testing me since I was about 40 for prostate cancer. The more common age for testing is 50 (unless there is a history of the disease in the family). The dreaded DRE (Digital Rectal Examination), whilst unpleasant, takes only a minute and what's a minute of discomfort when it can prevent a serious illness? It was all just a matter of course. I would be out of there as soon as possible and on my way to the gym, good health and wellbeing. I didn't realise then that this day would change my life forever, especially hearing my doctor's slightly concerned voice informing me about my enlarged prostate.

'Probably nothing to worry about,' he said, 'but worth obtaining a PSA reading.'

It could have been any one of a number of things but because of my young age, prostate cancer was considered highly unlikely. A PSA?

Upon enquiry I was told it was a Prostate Specific Antigen test which measures the level of Prostate Specific Antigen (PSA) in the blood and it can help to diagnose prostate disease. I felt embarrassed that I didn't even know what it was.

Arriving home, I started thinking about the PSA result. It was probably nothing to worry about and my understanding was that prostate cancer mostly affected men in their 60s, 70s and upwards. There was no history in my family of prostate cancer, although my biological father died at the age of 23, and both my grandfathers had died in their early 50s, so I guess we didn't really know all the facts from either side of the family.

When I arrived home, I rang my good friend Chris. He'd researched an enlarged prostate on Google and learned that it could be attributed to many things other than cancer. What a relief! I could stop worrying.

Still, I was distracted all week, both at home and at work. I spoke to my dear friend Mirna at work one afternoon; she is also a counsellor, as many of my friends are. I told her of my test and my alarm at what the results might indicate. It wasn't till many months later that she told me that I had appeared different that day and that, despite her reassurances, it seemed that somewhere deep inside of me I had already guessed that I had cancer. She had heard it in my voice. I already knew.

I had to go back to my GP a week later to obtain the results of my blood tests. I had traversed this path many times over the years, never worrying. That said, I was a bit uneasy this time.

My GP ushered me into his office, gave me all the blood results (which were all excellent), leaving the PSA until the very end. It was 5.9. He mentioned again that, while there was probably nothing to worry about, it would be advisable to see a urologist and seek their professional opinion. He knew I was anxious - he could see it, hear it in my voice. He knew me well enough.

I immediately made an appointment with a highly recommended urologist for a few days later. He was a serious man; it went with the territory. He performed another DRE. More unpleasantness. His voice showed some concern; there was a rough patch on the surface of the prostate. A highish PSA, an enlarged prostate and a rough surface - three things not in my favour. I felt sick. The doctor suggested another PSA test, as well as a biopsy, which was scheduled for early in December. This was to be day surgery. The doctor said that it was a simple procedure, no pain, but there would be some interference to the prostate and this would cause my semen to become bloodied and that I would ejaculate what looked like dark brown diesel oil. The day of my biopsy came and went smoothly.

It was Sunday night, 6 December 2009. I drank a couple of glasses of red wine, mindlessly watched television, and contemplated the next day when I would probably receive my biopsy results. The phone suddenly rang. It was about 8.30 pm. It was my urologist.

His voice was clear and serious. There had been thirty cores taken and only one core had shown to be positive for cancer - a very small tumour right in the centre of the prostate.

'Will I die?' I asked, matter of factly.

'No,' the answer came back quickly and firmly. 'We have caught it early, it's very small and it's right in the middle, not towards the outer shell of the prostate – which is good news.'

I couldn't think properly. He relayed some of the facts and statistics to me. I found it hard to concentrate, maybe due to my anxiety or the wine or a combination of both. He wanted to see me later in the week after I had digested the news. I booked an appointment for Thursday night, 10th December.

The few days after receiving the news, I surprisingly felt good. The cancer was treatable and beatable. They could cut it out of my prostate and I would return to good health. Nothing will have changed – just a small hiccup in the bigger scheme of things.

My doctor's appointment was late at night. My dear dad came with me. I had been told that it is always useful to take someone with you as an extra pair of ears and an attitude of greater objectivity. He was the perfect person to accompany me. He is very methodical, sensible and smart, and he listens attentively. Together we had prepared a series of questions that we needed to ask – what were my treatment options being the first.

The hospital floor was in darkness except for one small light at the end of the corridor. It looked so gloomy and ominous. The doctor welcomed us in. My father and I sat down and listened to the barrage of options that lay before me and all the associated facts and data that come with a diagnosis of prostate cancer – radiotherapy, brachytherapy, surgery, prostatectomy, the Da Vinci robot, PSA scores, Gleason scores, American results, Australian results, figures, data, impotence, incontinence. Facts, facts and more facts. The good news was that he felt he could get rid of the cancer (the number one concern!), but the bad news was that there were side-effects of each of the various approaches.

After surgery, for example, there would be no semen or ejaculate present, the seminal vesicles would be removed along with the prostate and there could be a 50% chance of impotence. I was told I would still be able to have an orgasm, though. *Huh? That didn't make sense!* There was so much my head was trying to comprehend. Where was the social worker to deal with the emotional fallout of this conversation? I felt scared, bewildered, overwhelmed and faint. *Was this really happening?* I stared into space and saw the doctor's lips moving, although no sound emerged. I think he decided that we had spoken for long enough and that he didn't want to overload me with any more information (*too late for that!*), so he welcomed me back to discuss and review the options at a later date. Think things over. The good thing, according to the doctor, was that we had plenty of time; we didn't have to rush.

Just prior to leaving, I asked the doctor for a private word. My father vacated the room and went and sat in the waiting room outside. Tears welled up in my eyes.

'Doctor, I am 46, a single, gay man who hasn't yet found his life partner. This news is devastating to me. What happens to these men who have poor outcomes after treatment and end up both incontinent and impotent?'

He looked at me and said the scariest word in the world to me: 'Depression.'

'What happens to their sex life?'

The doctor referred to the fact that sex can become less spontaneous and might need to be more planned. One can take medication (Viagra or Cialis, of course), a self-administered injection, an implant that costs $11,000, and the incontinence (whilst unlikely for my age) could be managed using incontinence pads.

Really, these are my options? I felt so old. 'Can I speak to a social worker or is there a support group I can attend?'

The doctor advised me that there was no social worker and the support group was mainly comprised of much older men in their 60s and up and that I may feel a sense of alienation within the group given my younger age. He certainly wasn't recommending it.

'Will I still feel an attraction towards men without having my prostate?' I asked.

'It will be like admiring a picture,' came back the reply.

A picture! It sounds like I will be admiring the fucking Mona Lisa.

I wanted to ask so many more questions, intimate ones about my sex life and yet I felt awkward doing so. I looked at his photo of he and his wife and children, beautifully framed and so proudly placed on his desk.

What about anal sex? Penetrative sex? Receptive sex? How will the absence of semen affect my orgasm? How can you reach orgasm with a flaccid penis? Will I still be a sexual man? Will I feel attractive to other men?

These were all such personal questions interconnected with my identity and I needed answers to reduce my anxiety and yet I just couldn't bring myself to ask them. I felt embarrassed revealing myself to this man and caught up in a heterosexist world, just like I always had.

I left the hospital and said goodbye to my dad. I had arranged to meet Chris afterwards to discuss my results. I was totally wired. Chris and I walked and talked around the block, across the street, around the park, back around the block – me leading the way, Chris following me wherever I decided to go, both conversationally and geographically.

What did all this news mean for my identity, my masculinity, my ego, my sexuality, my love life, my lust life, my relationships, my future? Why couldn't I handle this more maturely, confidently, like other men? Why couldn't I take it in my stride, methodically, like my father would have instead of feeling so hysterical about it? I was so ashamed of myself. Why was I creating such a big deal out of this? The doctor could save my life and rid the cancer from my body before it spread. Surely this was the most important point; to be cancer-free. What about impotence, though? And the idea of being incontinent simply made me feel so much older than my 46 years.

My mother had not been well and had been in hospital having complicated back surgery. I had been in the exact same hospital at the same time having my biopsy, just two floors below. The family and I had not told her of my cancer diagnosis as we did not want her to worry and wanted her to recover fully from her operation first. She would find out soon enough, although it was not a conversation I was looking forward to as I knew it would really upset her. The day came a week later and I asked Dad to explain the diagnosis to her and what it meant. I knew I would cry when I saw her after she had digested the news. I have really only ever seen my mother cry once before: first, when I told her I was gay, and again now, when I told her that I had cancer.

Christmas approached rapidly. The stores were becoming overstocked with possible gifts for friends and relatives alike. Christmas trees adorned the shop windows. People were happy, celebrating, drinking and feasting and going to parties, whilst I socially retreated into an internal world of fear. I didn't want to die of cancer, nor did I want to die from being depressed and unable to live my life fully and happily. I had suffered from depression twice before and this had been a major upset and embarrassment for me. There is still a lot of stigma attached to depression. Feelings of being weak, thinking negatively, not being manly and not coping were all ideas that I identified strongly with. I felt worthless and the future looked grim. Who would want to be with someone who couldn't perform sexually was a serious question to me. In my world there was so much emphasis placed on one's sexual performance.

Jan and Margaret are two very dear work colleagues who probably felt the major part of my emotional collapse. I went into work on this particular day, having decided that I would need some time out and would not be able to attend to the volume of marking that I had to complete over the Christmas period. Telling Margaret what had transpired in the last two weeks, I broke down. I described my experience of the last few weeks using catastrophic words like 'devastated' and 'gutted', not knowing what the future would now hold for a single 46-year-old gay guy looking for love in this big city. This was uppermost in my thoughts, as was that fearful word: *depression*. I explained to my dear friend Jan that a life living with depression was a life not worth living. I had been there before, I had seen what it had done to my family, and the thought became intrusive and dark. To me, this would be worse than dying of cancer. Margaret and Jan were both marvellous; they listened to me, comforted me. They just didn't know what to say to keep me from crying. I was inconsolable.

I had friends coming to stay with me over Christmas, two wonderful friends, Mary and Anthony, and my twin goddaughters. Telling my friends that I had cancer was the next thing to manage. It was like 'coming out' all over again. I felt so ashamed. I admitted to them in my kitchen one morning how I felt the cancer was my fault, my doing. I had lived a fairly reckless life in my twenties and thirties, smoking a lot of pot, drinking copiously most weekends, eating lots of red meat and not enough fish, not exercising, smoking cigarettes for eighteen years, and having many sexual partners (albeit I still practised safe sex). I felt remorseful that I had not led a healthier life when I had the opportunity to do so.

Why have I been so stupid? What have I done to deserve this? Is this some kind of bad karma? Had all my worries about being gay finally resulted in a build-up of tension and anxiety and stress resulting in prostate cancer? It's all been my doing!

Somehow these thoughts of shame and embarrassment and guilt had paralleled with my 'coming out' experience when I was 37. Back then I had felt ashamed of my attraction to men, and that somehow it had all been my fault and that I hadn't tried hard enough to become a heterosexual man. I had felt disgusted with who I was. My Catholic upbringing was hard at work on my fragile psyche. My darkest memories are of having undergone aversive therapy in the mid 1980s at the age of 22 under the specialist 'care' of a psychiatrist, who had tried to make me straight. I had actually agreed to receive electric shocks to accompanying thoughts of having sex with men to try to make me straight, have my family be ultimately proud of me, have society approve of me, and be able to then go on to live the life that I had been groomed for; marrying and having children. I knew that the aversive therapy was a totally absurd 'cure' but I was so desperate to conform. Those months were humiliating. I felt like a laboratory rat, engaged in a psychological experiment that was utterly futile and painful. Physically, it was unpleasant; psychologically, it was devastating. I felt scarred and have ever since. My self-esteem had always been low and continued to be for most of the next twenty years of my life. I feel so sad as I reflect on this period of my life.

My friends stayed over the lead-up to Christmas and I moved to my parent's home, seeking refuge from the world. I started to see my old counsellor again, a psychologist who was to become a major part of my life over the next six months. She had run my 'coming-out' group when I was 33 – when I had just started to come out to myself and accept who I was. She is an amazing woman, highly skilled, compassionate, trustworthy, good-humoured and totally committed to her clients and her profession. She is one of the nicest people I have ever met. The day that I went to see her, I announced in a lethargic voice that I had been diagnosed with prostate cancer. I explained my feelings of anxiety around my future, and my feelings of depression returning that she had worked tirelessly with me on years before. She heard me and empathised with me – which was so important – and she helped me to connect with another young, gay, male survivor of prostate cancer to talk with him about his experience with cancer and how he had managed, despite his results of surgery not being that successful. I needed this connection desperately; I needed to ask all my personal questions to someone who was young, gay and had travelled similar terrain. I needed hope and reassurance that I would be okay. I felt that he would understand and he did and I felt remarkably better after my conversation with him. This connection seemed such an essential part of my mental and emotional coping.

The weeks went on and I continued to feel dazed. I became totally obsessed with my cancer and the possible side effects of the various treatment options. The term's teaching work had come to completion two weeks before, which meant that I didn't have to manage my teaching load, marking, nor any other work-related duties. We had holidays until early January, which gave me time to concentrate on myself – probably not such a good thing, as I had way too much time on my hands. I had been told by the doctors to review the literature on prostate cancer, watch some DVDs on the topic, read information and pamphlets, talk to survivors, ask questions and seek answers, practice meditation and get some exercise. The literature unavoidably concentrated on heterosexual couples in their later years, discussing their situation. Even the text of talk to your 'partner' rather than wife was laden with heterosexual images. I felt so alienated from the support resources and material. *Where are my resources? Why aren't I included? What about me?*

I received a second opinion from another specialist in the field that reinforced that the most suitable option for me, given my age, tumour size and Gleason score of seven was the radical prostatectomy using the Da Vinci robot and nerve-sparing techniques. Prostate cancer normally strikes men in their 60s and up. Most men will die with prostate cancer and not of it. In younger men it can be a faster-growing cancer. My expected lifespan was longer and radiotherapy carried long-term side effects of erectile difficulties and the possibility of return of the cancer in areas located next to the damaged area, such as the bladder and the bowel. I desperately wanted to talk to other men who were young and to hear of stories with positive outcomes. Everything so far seemed so pessimistic. I wished there had been a cancer support group for young, gay men. Unfortunately, I was told there was no such thing available.

My stepbrother and his husband live in Wellington, New Zealand. I love them and have a special relationship with them. They demonstrated their support for me by linking me up with a friend of theirs who was the same age as me, gay, and who had had external beam radiation a few years before. I rang him and talked endlessly to him over the phone, asking all those personal questions I needed answers to, seeking his recommendations, hearing his choices and their subsequent results. There is one sure thing when discussing prostate cancer that you can't avoid: you connect immediately with the heart of someone's being, the essence of being a man, their sexuality and who they are.

My urologist also kindly sent me a letter recommending that I speak to another man who was younger than me (in his 30s) and had recovered amazingly well from his surgery. Within one week of his surgery his erectile functioning and continence had returned. This was highly irregular as I had heard that it can take up to three years for functioning to resume and in most cases it would never return to its full potency – if at all. This was what I needed to hear: a positive story from a younger man. Over the next few months I was to hear a range of stories from friends and relatives. So many people had stories linked to a friend or relative that they knew. There were some wonderful stories and some awful ones. I heard the difficulty in making choices for many men. This was certainly a unique issue of this particular type of cancer. One had options to consider, unlike other cancers, which did not.

It was six months before I made up my mind to choose the surgery option, an agonising six months of obsession and high levels of anxiety. I had been unsuccessfully trying to adopt the watchful waiting option. The tumour was minute, I reminded myself. I was so scared of losing my potency and continence that I would do anything that prevented the treatment, despite the incessant nagging from my family to have the surgery. Everyone talked about the Big C, but I was worried about the Big I and its impacts on my mental health. My psychologist was simply amazing through this period, seeing me weekly and sometimes even daily. She helped me place things in perspective, talking about more positive possibilities, challenging my negative, catastrophic thinking and helping me relax and stay calm, reframing things and helping me create meaning out of what I was going through. She drew attention to my strengths and resources and she acknowledged my many support systems.

It was now February and I was back working, albeit not being fully present and engaged in what I was doing, a couple of times having panic attacks in the middle of my classes. It was a bumpy six months of tossing around the options, indecision, talking to people, doctors, sexual health rehabilitation specialists and patients.

The final clincher for me, though, was when the urologist said that if I was his brother, he would be advising that I act now and not leave it any longer. This turned out to be magical encouragement as, unbeknownst to me, the cancer had started to spread within the prostate. I went to bed that night, thinking I would never forgive myself if I waited any longer and they had found that the cancer had broken through the shell of the prostate and had spread to other nearby organs, the lymph system, the bones. I rang at 9.00 am the next day, and made my appointment for surgery the first thing on the morning of 5 July 2010. Enough waiting; I was ready. My family and friends were both relieved and delighted, especially my dear mum and dad.

Jacki is one of my closest friends and has supported me so totally throughout this incredible journey. Given my current circumstances, I was about to lose my prostate and hence my semen and capacity to ejaculate, she asked me whether I had thought of sperm donation prior to my operation. It suddenly dawned on me that this would be the last possible opportunity for me to become a father. (I have since learned that sperm can be drained from the testes as another viable alternative to having children.) This was a loss that I believed I had dealt with many years before upon coming out as a gay man, the prospect that I probably would never become a parent and now that whole idea resurfaced and I found myself deliberating over the possibility yet again. *Do I want to become a father? A sperm donor?* I pondered this thought for another month, the time ticking by and the operation now due in only five days on Monday morning at 8.00 am. I had the weekend to decide my fate on this topic. I had decided that there would be no harm in freezing my sperm. I made my appointment the following day to go in to the clinic, enabling parenting choice for my future or the possibility of donation at some later date. I was told that the cut-off date for donation was fifty years of age. I had just scraped in.

I made my way to the clinic, completed the paperwork and sighted the young men in the waiting room. I was taken to my private room, given a plastic bottle and my attention turned towards the numerous *Penthouse* magazines on the small table in the middle of the room. *Great!* There was a TV for viewing the pornography. *This is surreal.* I was so very anxious – anxious about the impending operation, anxious about 'performing' with this very tight deadline, anxious about the whole idea of becoming a parent. Needless to say my anxiety won over my ability to perform the required task and yet again a huge feeling of shame and failure took over me. I was angry with myself for my procrastination over the last month making me feel so powerless to the impending deadline. I left hurriedly in a daze of confusion and said goodbye to my final chance to become what I had always been groomed for – a father. I was devastated.

The day came for surgery and I was on edge. I showered using the disinfectant soap that they had given me to use, scrubbing myself vigorously. Dad and I bickered in the morning. Mum said goodbye. This was so very hard on her, the thought of one of her three children facing a serious operation.

We arrived at the hospital early. I was ushered to another level where I waited to be told what to do. I filled out more forms and papers, changed into the hospital gown, and lay on the bed that would soon wheel me down to the hospital operating room. Then something quite amazing happened. The nerves disappeared, the anxiety drained from my body and I felt completely calm. I guess I couldn't do anything now to change my mind. I felt I had made the right decision with the surgery and I would hope for the very best in terms of my outcomes. It was now beyond my control and up to a higher power to help me. I am not a particularly religious man and yet I found myself talking to a higher power to keep me safe and look after me from here. The nurses came to wheel me down to the operating room, Dad was at my bedside.

'I love you,' I said to him and then they wheeled me away.

The surgery went for about three hours and there were two surgeons and an anaesthetist present. I woke up in my room afterwards and the doctor came in to see me. He said that the operation had gone very well. They had removed the prostate gland and seminal vesicles and he thought that he had managed to successfully spare the nerves that surrounded the prostate, a difficult and tricky procedure. My head rested back on my pillow with a huge feeling of relief. How great to hear such news! The cancerous prostate was gone. I guess the next thing was to wait until my body started to heal itself; my erections would hopefully return and my incontinence would disappear.

I spent four days lying in that bed in the hospital room, catheter in place, uncomfortable, drained, and tired. I felt like I was 100. The physiotherapist had me walking pretty quickly and when I asked my friend Tom to walk me down the corridor and back it was like doing the Boston marathon. Tom is also known for being a tremendous 'foodie' and good cook. Unbeknownst to me, he had prepared 14 gourmet meals and deposited them in my freezer to await my return home a few weeks later. This had been such a generous and practical gift that I really valued.

My recovery at home went tremendously well, especially upon hearing the news that the final biopsy result was that the cancer looked as if it had been contained within the shell of the prostate. There would be no need for radiation treatment. I experienced three weeks of incontinence and only one major mishap when I wet the bed. I was so relieved to have the catheter out, literally in a one-second pull-out motion by the nurse. It was also about three weeks into my recovery when I awoke in the early hours of the morning to find and feel an outstanding erection. I smiled and jumped out of bed and looked at myself naked in the mirror. I was both overwhelmed and excited. I was potent and after only three weeks! I had prepared myself for a three-year wait – if at all. I was so relieved! It seems nearly embarrassing wishing so much onto my erectile return but it was a big thing for me, especially being single and reliant on a more casual sex life where performance is considered so paramount.

I spent the next few weeks recuperating at my parents' home, being cared for and kept in a cosy cocoon against the harshness of the real world outside. My dad was such an amazing support to me; he looked after me, supplying me with comforting foods and our ritual of a glass of wine and the occasional spirits upon dinner time. My mum supported me in baking me my favourite roasts and dinners, which filled me with an endless supply of TLC. Needless to say, I put on ample kilos during my home stay. I think we were all relieved.

I went back to work after three weeks, which was way too early. I should have given it at least another six weeks to fully recover. I was anxious to return to work for as a sole trader I am not paid if I am not working, only I had a panic attack in the classroom and had to leave fairly quickly. I needed to have another week off work to settle myself and land properly. I never told my students what was happening except that I had needed to have some surgery for health-related concerns. They didn't ask any questions. I was back on deck a week later, four weeks after the operation and dancing around my classroom like nothing had happened.

One year after the surgery, I spoke to a social worker in Melbourne who worked for the Cancer Council there. She advised me of a pilot group that was starting up in Sydney to explore the needs of gay and bisexual men who have a prostate cancer diagnosis. Coincidentally, I had also seen an ad in the gay press for this group looking for men to come forward with their stories. I rang and spoke to the organiser and social worker Greg straight away and put my name down to attend the pilot group which would run for three consecutive Tuesdays. This was to be an invaluable part of my healing, creating meaning out of what had been a difficult time in my life; I knew this also as a counsellor – creating meaning for clients out of their experience is an important part of their therapeutic recovery. I also remember Mirna saying a year earlier that maybe I would one day work in this arena and she was right!

The three workshops were run professionally by Greg, a very experienced social worker in the area of men's health. Greg is also gay and had experiences with his own type of cancer: leukaemia. He collated data about our experiences through three stages: diagnosis, treatment and after care. The three weeks went by very quickly and I met a wonderful group of 15 gay/bisexual identifying men all with interesting stories to tell. I was the second youngest in the group and found some solace talking to the other young males in the group. Most participants were single except for two or three – which I personally found an interesting statistic – and there were a range of different personalities and cultures in the room. I felt that I was contributing to something quite special during this period and eagerly and vocally added my thoughts and shared my experiences. We looked at how things could be improved from a gay man's perspective as we had been the forgotten group. Now I felt included. I was finding my voice in trying to shape things differently for future gay and bisexual men going through the challenges accompanying a prostate cancer diagnosis.

The Shine-A-Light group in Sydney was born in 2010 and has been running every first Saturday of every month, for three years at the ACON offices in Surry Hills. The group is an open group for men affected by prostate cancer – who identify as gay or bisexual – and their partners. I have often been asked why do we need a separate group for gay and bisexual men and my answer is to provide a safe place for these men to discuss their concerns and their sexual lives free from any heterosexist norms, judgements and prejudices, which many gay and bisexual men have encountered at some point throughout their lives. It is a non-judgemental space to discuss our thoughts, share our emotions, how we have coped or possibly haven't. Our group is open to people who have had all possible treatment options and who are dealing with their various impacts on mind, body and soul. We have a range of speakers to talk about things like diet and nutrition, surgeons, urologists, sexual rehabilitation specialists, educators in alternative sexual practice and more. We attend to the needs of different people in the room as best as we can. We laugh and we cry. The main thing is about connecting with each other and sharing stories, highs and lows, ups and downs, with like-minded people. It is a chance to share knowledge and support each other. It is a social opportunity that gives added meaning to those on this journey, helping others through a frightening time in their lives. It is about making friends.

I am 50 now and another milestone and a new chapter in my life has begun. Life seems amazingly good. I have balance restored. I still see a counsellor every week for added support. I have meaning in my life; I have become an ambassador to the Prostate Cancer Foundation of Australia. I have made some marvellous friends from the Shine-a-Light group. I attend training days to improve the functioning of our support group. I have had a role to play in the development and distribution of new resources for gay and bisexual men. I feel included in the support material and resources available to gay and bisexual men and feel I have contributed my voice to the wellbeing of these men who are in various stages of dealing with their prostate cancer diagnoses. I remain a lecturer and have a counselling practice based in Redfern. I provide support to many men, both gay and straight, of all ages and cultural backgrounds and hear of their experiences, the good and the not so good. I feel relieved and grateful for my good health. My last PSA, which I now only have to have every six months, was 0.01. I play tennis once a week and I have a fitness instructor. My brother and his wife have since had three beautiful children. I now have two nephews and another niece. I am still single and I lead a happy life.

I want to finish by saying thank you to my surgeon who did such a brilliant job on all three fronts of removing the cancer and restoring me back to full continence and near 100% potency levels and to all my wonderful family and friends who have helped and supported me on my journey and who have played an integral part in my recovery and in my life.

My Prostate Journey

Bruce Lamb

When I was 60-years-old, I asked a GP for a check-over so he ordered full bloods. I had done the same thing when I was 50.

Results came back good except for a PSA of 13. I was referred to a specialist clinic at Redcliffe Hospital. I had some discussion with the specialist who presented my options to me – watch and wait, radiation treatment, or surgery.

The emotion of hearing his message rattled my cage a lot and I really did not know which way to turn. The urologist suggested I talk with the Radiation Oncologist.

Oncologist? Hearing that, it really hit home.

7.08.07

A TRUSS biopsy showed 20% cancer (Right Apex Lateral) and Gleason 4+3=7 T2.

14.11.07

Had discussion with Radiation Doctor. She was very abrupt and I felt very pushed to accept. I tentatively agreed to the radiation. I wished to have further discussion with the doctor about the procedure but I was unable to contact her. I made several calls and the nurse who answered said I could ask the doctor on the day. I did this and was then blasted for wasting her time.

22.1.08

Signed the papers for the surgical procedure.

8.4.08

Had all the usual CT scan of abdomen and pelvis bone scan for checks the cancer had not metastasized.

15.4.08

Bi-Lateral Pelvic Lymph Dissection + Radical Prostatectomy (non-nerve sparing) at Redcliffe Hospital. Surgeon Dr J, 8.43 am – 13.24 pm.

Day 1 Post-Surgery

Came into ward in AF (Atrial Fibrillation, where the heart goes out of normal sinus rhythm). It makes one feel very weak, but it also means that the heart is not delivering full pressure to all the organs. I have had this condition for many years and was on Beta Blockers to keep my heart rhythm stable. I told staff this happens all the time and lasts a few hours to a few days. The nurses were angels and did everything they could to make me comfortable. I must confess to feeling very vulnerable, but was very assured by one particular nurse named Jenny.

Day 2

Doing well, looking well, and drains were removed.

First few days were normal. Expected (by Friday they were talking about going home) recovery except that I had a large scrotum (ten centimetres reported in nurse's notes) and, over the next week, it went through many (black and blue) colours.

I was not using the 'pain management button' and the pain crew were surprised that I was not needing extra shots. I had no pain to speak of but they left the pain management button there for a few days anyway.

My main aggravation was the catheter – not comfortable at all. My legs started to swell – in particular my left one was like a tree trunk – and my stomach was growing.

Day 4

Had a cry, not because of any pain, but as a kind of a release of nervous tension. I think it may be like a mother after she has had a baby; your body has had a massive interruption and this is a reaction to it. Anyway, because my Atrial Fibrillation had not ceased and I was not feeling well, I was transferred to a medical ward. There was a need for my heart to be monitored full time and, if it did not change, maybe my heart would have to be stopped and restarted to get it back into rhythm.

The nursing staff wanted to look at my wounds, as they did not see the surgery. One nurse said I should photograph my scrotum for memories but this is not really something you want in the family album so we decided not to.

Day 6

In the early hours of morning, the nurse came and asked how I felt; I said like a hand was resting on my chest. She told me, 'That is the hand of God', and that I had returned to normal rhythm. The next day I was returned from the medical ward to the surgical ward.

Day 7

A day I will never forget, as with most abdominal surgery you get wind in your body cavity so I had a need to pass some wind. My logic said it would be best to let gravity assist here so I stood up.

Here we go.

I got rid of some wind but the effort blew open about a third of the stitches. I had a half-circle of fluid on the floor in front of me. I called the nurse who promptly put me on my bed. The doctor was called and he said, 'Believe it or not, this is good.' Didn't look it from where I stood, but it had gotten rid of that build-up of fluid in my stomach.

It turned out my lymph nodes had not sealed after the pre-op biopsy they had had to do before the deep surgery. Because of the discharge I had a blood transfusion that day, too (two units).

Day 8

Because of the fluid still in my body, they needed to put some drainers to allow it out. By good fortune, I had one of the best doctors in the state of Queensland for inserting drainers. To get complete accuracy, a CT scan was used to guide the doctor to the right spot. Eventually, almost a litre of fluid was drained.

Day 9

My stomach was smaller now. Still worried about swollen legs, but I was assured they would go down.

Day 11

All surgical staples were removed (should have been only half of them but okay).

Day 13

I left hospital on 28th April. They showed my wife how to dress the wound but she felt it was beyond her, so the local nurse came to dress the wound daily. I had a catheter in for two more weeks.

1st May

Had a cystogram to check healing process.

Continence rehab was not too bad once catheter was removed. I had a bottle by the bed and over a week or so was able to make it to the toilet to release. Wore pads for a few weeks and progressively slowed to a drip when stressed. Otherwise, good.

Normal post-op treatment once you leave hospital would be to visit the hospital several times to see if you were recovering continence and some pelvic floor exercises would be practiced while there. Because my home was two hours from the hospital, (I had moved house from the time of consultation to surgery) I was referred to my local hospital for some physio and there I did pelvic floor exercises, which were checked with an ultrasound machine to ensure I was doing them correctly.

The main complaint was there was no real information about the procedure and the decision-making of what to have. I had to search the internet myself and sort through a myriad of information from here and America before I could decide.

I am now a volunteer with Cancer Council Tasmania to help others who are going through what I did. I also inform first-year medical students how I felt as a patient.

Information is much more available now.

Ode to Prostates

Judith O'Malley-Ford

At the beginning
　of June, At 12 minutes
　to noon, or perhaps 11 to three,
　　　at a place of your choosing,
　　　without ever losing
　　　　the fact that
　　　　　　it's coffee
　　　　　　or tea.
I'm just a GP,
　　　but not like on TV,
　　　　　I am writing a
　　　　　book about men.
　　　　　Their prostates are prone
　　　　　to a moan and a groan
　　　　　'cos they're afflicted
　　　　again, and again.
　With their health
　down the drain,
　I'll say
　　　　it again,
　　　　They need
　to take
　　　　stock

of their senses,
but I'm not here
to trick you,
To treat you
or trip you,
I'm happy just
minding my tenses.
So here let us boast,
And let's drink
a toast,
With coffee
or tea it's all right.
With delusions of grandeur,
I'm glad
that I found
ya',
under cover of
darkness
at
night.

Against All Odds:
A Positive Story From a
Prostate Cancer Survivor

Steve Radojevic

Just a few words about myself – I'm married to Heather, my gorgeous wife of twenty-nine years; we have two beautiful daughters we are very proud of: Jade is 22 and Lauren is 20. I have a wonderful mum, Tania, who is only 72, and thinks I'm pretty special (but, of course, all mums think that of their sons). Then there's my loving sister, Anita, and her family. I'm also blessed with fabulous extended family and friends.

In May 2005 I had just turned 44 and was feeling unusually tired and knew something wasn't quite right. I went to my long-time GP and asked him to run some blood tests. He asked me whether he should run one for prostate whilst he was at it and I said yes. I used to get up at night to go to the toilet and when it was cold it seemed like I was going more than all the other guys at work during the day.

A week later I got a call from my GP asking me to come in and see him. He told me the news could be very bad – my PSA was 8.1 and for someone my age the upper limit should be 2.5. My GP came around the desk and gave me a hug and then referred me to a urologist. Within weeks I had a biopsy and, subsequently, I was told that seven of the ten hits were cancerous and I was in for a fight to beat the cancer.

Over the following weeks I rang the Cancer Council to find out exactly what my chances of survival were. I was unpleasantly surprised to find that, statistically, I had no chance of beating the cancer, given my age, PSA and biopsy results.

I'm going to die, I thought.

I made up my mind that I would go through the process of whatever was recommended and that at least no one could say I gave up. I consciously decided to keep things in perspective. I had had so many wonderful experiences in my life; it was time for me to handle adversity being mindful of others rather than it being about me. I can't begin to imagine how difficult and scary the experience was going to be for my wife, and two daughters, who were only 13 and 11 years old at the time.

Further to consultation with my urologist and a number of trips to the Peter MacCallum Cancer Centre, it was decided that a radical prostatectomy would be the best bet. The operation was unsuccessful in that the cancer had gone beyond the prostate and my PSA was still traceable. Further consultation with my urologist led to me being referred to a radiologist that led to seven weeks of radiation. The radiologist said, 'This is your last chance.' He asked me if I knew what that meant.

I knew.

Eight months after I finished the radiation I was told that was it, that the radiation had not worked and my PSA was rising again. He raised the possibility of having chemotherapy and I declined. That day he told me I would not recover, my wife and I walked from his office and my wife said, 'I don't care what he says you are going to get better.'

I spoke with my GP friend about timing for making DVDs for my daughters' 21st birthdays, weddings, etc. He said it was a good idea to get them done, you never know how quickly you can go, given that the younger you are when diagnosed with prostate cancer the more aggressive the cancer is. I was told hormone therapy may help – come back in six months to see where your score has got to.

That was in December 2006.

Five years before I found out I had cancer my dad was diagnosed with cancer and he found out he was going to die from it. He was devastated but I told him to be grateful for all the wonderful things that had happened in his life and how lucky his life had been compared to so many others. He was 61 years old and said it was easy for me because I wasn't the one dying. He died six weeks later. Well, now it was my turn to walk the talk. I truly feel I have had a wonderful life and if it was shorter than some others so be it. Getting old has its downsides as well. I often joked that I was getting bored with life. Time to move on.

Up to this stage, my GP, urologist, radiologist, and oncologist all dismissed my ideas of changing my diet or any form of complementary healing. In Europe, most cancer specialists recommend a visit to a naturopath, meditation and working on positive emotions (as a minimum) to boost your immune system to help fight the cancer.

When I was first diagnosed, Mark Kennedy, a friend and local GP, encouraged me to explore other options to complement conventional medical practices. He is a man I have a lot of respect for and now I had some added motivation to give integrative or alternative healing concepts a serious go. Let's face it: my health was charting south at a rapid rate so, if I didn't change something, I knew where I was heading.

I was also hounded by family and friends to try everything so I thought, *Why not?* and decided to give it my best shot to stay alive as long as possible. I read a book called *How to Fight Prostate Cancer and Win*. I also read another book written by Ian Gawler, who had beaten cancer by using his mind and changing his diet. I was introduced to meditation, reiki, naturopaths and an array of alternative healing methods that I would have laughed at previously.

A lot of the books I read were consistent in that their evidence substantiated that clear, positive, hopeful, optimistic thoughts – even when there is no basis for these – are a powerful medicine in healing. What we feel, think, say and do has a profound influence on our mental, physical and spiritual health.

Everyone knows about the placebo effect. The University of Tennessee for Health Science conducted a study that gave people suffering from chronic pain a pill that would make them feel better. It was, in fact, just a sugar pill. Forty-four percent felt better – by believing the pill was making them better actually made them feel better. If you realise how powerful your thoughts are you will never want to think a negative thought again. My goal was to only think positive thoughts, all the time!

I made up my mind I was going to keep enjoying and concentrating on living life. An *attitude of gratitude* was my catchcry. Whilst I'm here I want to appreciate the wonderful people and opportunities surrounding me. It also meant taking responsibility and ownership for my own recovery and having a fighting spirit. They say the best luck of all is the luck you make for yourself.

It was also at this time that I asked God for help. I asked him to help me stay around for awhile to help bring up my family. I asked for all the prayers and kind thoughts that were out there for me to give me strength to let me help other people. I have always said a prayer my whole life before falling asleep. Ninety-nine percent of the time, it was a prayer of thanks for the wonderful people in my life, or I would pray for other people who are sick or have died. I felt that I was so lucky that I shouldn't ask God for anything. It would be greedy. But the day I was told I was not going to get better was the same night I asked for an extension of life.

Well, go figure, the next time I went to the urologist – six months later – my PSA was untraceable. He said he couldn't explain it. I said that there was merit in all the things I had done. He asked me to explain what I had been doing and now he actually could see merit in some of the things I had done. My PSA is still untraceable. I have been told that I am in the clear now. My urologist previously dismissed my ideas of complementary healing, saying there was no scientific evidence of their success. Now he recommends some of the very things he had once dismissed. He and I spoke at the Victorian Prostate Cancer Conference in 2010. I was a guest speaker as someone who had survived against the odds and used an integrative approach to fighting cancer. My urologist was the next speaker and he spoke of the fact that he was my surgeon and urologist and that he had changed his mind about diet, positive thinking and taking steps to help your recovery. It was the best endorsement I could have had in front of a large audience mainly full of people who were looking to improve their chances of recovery.

I'd like to share with you the things I did/changed that may have helped me achieve a turnaround in results. There is a Chinese proverb I like that describes my change in behaviour: 'Only after you encounter affliction and adversity will you summon the mind of diligence.'

- **Naturopath**: They aim to identify how your enzymes are performing. They will make you do a liver function test that determines which nutrients are lacking in your body, then recommend vitamins and specific food to get you back into a healthy balance again. Make sure that you get your immune system right! The aim is to eliminate toxins from your body, then nourish it with food that is natural and healthy.
- **Tomato paste**: The little Leggo tubs are full of antioxidants. Prostate cancer is less prevalent in countries that eat a diet rich in tomato paste. The paste is much better for you than real tomatoes, because it is a concentrate. The secret ingredient is called lycopene.
- **Pumpkin seeds**: A small handful a day are excellent for your plumbing health.
- **Blueberries**: Full of antioxidants.
- **Filtered water**: Nikken PiMag Water System.

Healthy stuff

My top recommendations that keep coming up through all the success stories are as follows:

- **Selenium**: Mineral found in soils in countries where there are the lowest rates of cancer. Australian soil has little or no selenium, so this is well worth taking for minimising or keeping cancer away. Brazil nuts are a great source of selenium if you want to get your nutrients through food. Just have three or four brazil nuts a day.
- **Zinc**: Helps for healing. Also available through eating oysters, and pumpkin seeds.
- **Coenzyme Q10**: Tablet – spark plug nutrient for regenerating healthy cells.
- **Vitamin D3**: For Vitamin D deficiency. There is very strong evidence suggesting there is a relationship between people with prostate cancer and Vitamin D deficiency. During winter I take a tablet a day.
- **China White tea**: Strongest tea for fighting cancer from Leaf Tea shop 124 Ryrie Street, Geelong. The benefits of antioxidants in supporting our immune system are real.
- **Cholesterol**: I read that there may be evidence that higher cholesterol is a factor for PC. I have made an effort to lower mine.

Things to cut out

- Artificial sweeteners (carcinogenic), sugar, red meat as much as possible and dairy.

Food and nutrition does make a difference, no question. A study found that the incidence of PC in Japanese men skyrocketed after moving to America due to a change in diet. Do your own research.

Google 'Prostate cancer in native Japanese and Japanese–American' for a comprehensive study of dietary differences on prostatic tissue.

Psycho immunology is also something to consider. Some can find it personally challenging or confronting, but it is going to get bigger over time. It proposes that psychological wellbeing is very important. Your wellbeing is tied into you having positive emotions.

Illness may come from unresolved issues – guilt, anger, resentment, or fear of the future. We need to get our minds in a good place. Learn to forgive as quickly as possible. No question unreleased or stuck emotions can create physical blockages that manifest themselves through illness. Stress causes restriction to blood flow and energy and this will only feed cancer. I believe that stress – emotional blockages along with an inadequate diet – were major factors in me getting cancer.

Do not underestimate the relationship between the mind and the body. The body behaves in the way the mind thinks so it is important to think healthy. Say to yourself 'Today my health is getting better', 'Today I am doing everything I can to make myself healthy again', 'Today every cell in my body responds positively to my positive mental images'. Doing this daily for a minute or two helps to align your brain into thinking yourself healthy. No question, positive thinking reduces stress and aids our immune system.

I went to see a lady called Jenny Limb in Queenscliff who specialises in healing people by working on their minds and realigning their thinking. In particular for me I had been told I wasn't going to get better and so Jenny had me visualising myself as healthy and cancer-free. It makes sense that your body responds to messages from your brain. Think healthy, be healthy.

- **Visualisation**: Visualise yourself being healthy. I use a common technique of imagining a white healing light coming into my body with my breath and clearing away the mutant cancer cells, leaving behind a healthy body. Again, remember this is important.

- **Our thoughts**: What we feel, think, say and do has a profound influence on our mental, physical and spiritual health.
- **Meditation:** A very good way to slow the mind down; it takes practice. You will always feel better after a session.
- **Reiki**: Hands-on healing. Very alternative. I have found it to be very effective and relaxing. The power of touch is not to be underestimated. Now being used in hospitals.
- **Sense of purpose**: Reason for living. Critical in healing, we need to have a reason to live – for family, looking forward to a big trip, the arrival of a grandchild, whatever it is, we need something to look forward to.
- **Read the Book**: *How to Fight Prostate Cancer and Win* by Ron Gellatley. Bestseller.

I love the following quote: 'Our lives are not determined by what happens to us, but by how we react to what happens. Not by what life brings to us but by the attitude we bring to life.'

I have changed; I eat a lot healthier; I have selenium, zinc, coenzyme Q10, fish oil, white tea, and pumpkin seeds most days. My diet is not perfect, although I have cut back on red meat and eliminated artificial sweeteners. I still have a drink, although not as much as I used to. I know my immune system is supported by the nutritional food I put into my body to nourish it. I still stress, but nowhere near as much as I did before. I meditate from time to time, I use healthy visualisation, I have reiki done on me, been to a homeopath, been to a naturopath, worked on my cholesterol, I and have resolved issues that have been with me since I was a kid – feelings of anger and resentment that were festering away. They are now occasional fleeting thoughts that don't take up brain space which is in short supply. I feel great most of the time and when I don't it is because I'm not getting enough rest or I am eating rubbish. I am back on track very quickly most of the time.

I haven't done everything that is out there – oxygen therapy, enemas, dental purification; I haven't gone for a super strict diet.

There is nothing really too sophisticated about what I do and I urge you to give it a go. I'm sure it has helped me in getting the great results I have been getting. Ask yourself, have you made changes? Have you taken ownership of this battle? Are you using some form of complementary medicine to support what is being recommended to you by your GP/urologist/radiologist/oncologist? In my opinion you should be.

Just as an aside I want to go on record as saying that getting cancer isn't the worst thing that could happen to you. We could have died from a heart attack and never had the chance to be told how much we are loved or to tell those we love how we feel about them. The sunsets are more beautiful. Friends are kinder. It has also given me the opportunity for tremendous personal growth. I have become better at saying no and focusing my time on what is important to me. It could all change for me at my next blood test; then I think to myself, *It is not the length of life but the depth of life that matters.* I've had wonderful experiences along the way that are worth three hundred years of living and I intend to have a few more before I go.

I have already made up my mind. I am going to try not to complain. I try to cultivate positive thinking in all aspects of my life, not just to enhance the quality of my life but also the lives of others – so we can have a positive effect on every receptionist, nurse, doctor, patient, carer, person we come into contact with and hopefully that will give them strength to pass it on in treating others with kindness and compassion. A positive attitude really can make dreams come true.

I'd like to thank you for giving me the opportunity to share my story. I extend best wishes to you and your families for today and the future.

Are We There Yet?

Danielle Burns

We first boarded this train about five years ago when at the ripe old age of 45 my husband, Ian, was diagnosed with prostate cancer.

Sitting in the specialist's waiting room, deep down we both knew that something big and shaky like this old red rattler was headed our way. Cancer was not new to us. We had watched Ian's lifelong hero, his dad, die from the same disease only a few years earlier. This had then been followed far too closely by his only sister's death at the age of 46 as a result of breast cancer and, after all that, his feisty mum had finally succumbed to the effects of throat cancer.

As we sat taking in the urologist's diagnosis, I decided we would not let cancer beat us this time. We would take a different approach. We'd been through it before and knew what to expect. We *could* cope. Then we'd both pull up our socks and get on with our lives. We'd beat this together and everything would be okay.

But when I looked up at Ian, it was clear he hadn't reached the same conclusion. Within that short space of time, he seemed to suddenly grow old. The colour drained from his face and the usual sparkle was gone from his eyes. When we got home, he didn't want to talk about the diagnosis or even look at any of the material we'd been given about his treatment options. Ian simply shut down.

To describe the next few days as a complete blur would be to grossly oversimplify things. We both wavered from anger, frustration and fear, to courage, strength and optimism. Either way, decisions had to be made. The shock of diagnosis is almost trumped by learning that the choice of treatment is left entirely to the patient. It's kind of like being thrown from a cliff while a passing stranger calls out, 'Aim for that flimsy net full of holes, or that rickety old swing bridge below!'

When we finally got around to discussing the information we'd been given, we found it was actually not very informative or even all that relevant. Most of it seemed aimed towards elderly patients. We decided that there must be better resources available somewhere. Ian called a PCA helpline listed on one of the brochures and was put in touch with a gentleman who had been through several similar procedures. Unfortunately, not only was he much older but he also had nothing enlightening or encouraging to offer. This experience only made Ian feel even more isolated and confused.

In an effort to try and take control of the situation I set about thoroughly researching the disease online. This provided me with a real purpose, as well as a much-needed sense of direction. I found so much out there on chat forums, websites and online support groups that Ian said later he felt overwhelmed with information. But, I was on a roll, trolling the internet till the wee early hours. I began compiling lists and comparing treatment options, including costs, duration, and also where and how each could be accessed in our region.

By the time we went back to the urologist, an informed decision had been made to undergo brachytherapy. Ian was referred to an eminent specialist in a large inner-city public hospital and we both attended the initial consultation with much trepidation. Just sitting in the waiting room watching cancer patients in varying degrees of ill-health brought to the surface our raw and recent memories of being in similar situations with missing family members. It was overwhelming.

However, we were soon reassured by the professionalism, experience and positivity of the entire medical team. They were very keen to offer this breakthrough treatment to a younger patient. Ian's procedure was viewed as an excellent opportunity for a case study. We both felt that his situation was finally being given the attention it deserved. We left filled with confidence in his outcome for the first time in weeks.

Of course, this is cancer we're talking about and it does have a nasty habit of changing course. Ian had required a TURP procedure prior to the treatment, which, in his case, significantly reduced the amount of prostate tissue available. This resulted in brachytherapy treatment being ruled out. Suddenly, we were back to that cliff-falling scenario and it seemed we were getting closer and closer to the edge.

After more research and a second surgical opinion, Ian finally underwent surgery to remove his prostate. He felt as though he'd spent so long in limbo and now he just wanted the cancer out of his body. We had different opinions on which method of surgery was appropriate but in the end, ignoring all my painstaking research, Ian followed his gut instinct and booked in for a laparoscopic radical prostatectomy.

His recovery from this operation was slow and painful. He had always had trouble sleeping and now couldn't even get comfortable sitting up on the couch. Ian also experienced lots of unexpected problems with the catheter and, as a result, was in constant agony. After this was removed, he gradually improved.

He tried really hard to just get up and get going again. Ian is and always has been a very practical, active person. He was never one to just sit back and relax but always kept busy with work, sport, family and a large circle of friends. But in those next few months Ian found it very difficult to get back into the swing of things.

It was tough to watch the man who had been my strength and inspiration for so many years become apprehensive and unsure. My reaction was to smother Ian with care and attention. Apparently there is a limit to the number of times one should ask, 'Are you okay?'

One of the biggest ongoing issues for him to cope with was incontinence. Ian had been asymptomatic when he was diagnosed, so he hadn't previously suffered any of these concerns, unlike most elderly patients. We'd researched the problem extensively and were convinced he would manage. Ian had consulted a specialised physiotherapist in the hope that the combination of exercise together with his pre-op fitness and relative youth, would ensure that bladder control wouldn't be as severe for him. But it wasn't to be. Although with his usual stubborn persistence, Ian somehow managed to cope. Most of the time, that is.

However, having now watched several friends go through this dreaded disease, I feel that nothing can adequately prepare a man for incontinence. Its effect on dignity and sense of masculinity amongst his peers should never be underestimated.

Impotence was to be the next big stumbling block. Although this is listed as only another side effect in all the literature, in reality – as most of us know – it's a totally separate condition. The consequences are even more far-reaching than incontinence and can be devastating for all involved. We had been together since we were teenagers, and I often joked that it was lucky we'd got started so early.

But in reality it was no laughing matter; it was an all-consuming problem for the both of us. We tried every method available, from medications to injections to pumps – most were ineffective, some were excruciatingly painful but Ian was still committed to finding a practical resolution. It was a huge obstacle in his recovery but he eventually accepted his limitations. This was to be the turning point. It meant we could both finally relax. We soon found different ways of doing things and let nature take its course.

The process of working through this delicate issue has somehow brought us even closer. We are both more aware and even more tolerant of the other's moods, needs and desires. It's a very different sort of intimacy to what we had in the past but then everything changes in time and ultimately the important thing is that we can still share our love for each other.

All throughout this time, we were also still trying to run our own business. With several projects underway and a dedicated team relying on us for work we really felt we had no other option. Ian was determined that everything would go on as it had before and that none of our clients, employees or subcontractors would be affected. My response was to pull on the old super-woman cape and try to take charge. Gradually, I took on more and more duties both at work and at home. It's amazing what you can achieve when the pressure is on.

Of course, there's also a limit to everything and eventually all this extra pressure took its toll on me too.

At the time, our three kids were teenagers – a time of life when they are much more interested in their peers than their parents' lives. But our kids also had to learn to cope with their own fears. They too had watched their extended family suffer the fatal effects of cancer.

Each of them handled the experience in their own way. Sometimes they took on extra responsibilities without being asked, while at other times they became frustrated with the added pressures of Dad being 'sick'. We tried to make sure they were all kept informed of their dad's progress and hopefully they always felt any question could be asked. We're really very proud of the way they rallied and helped each other through this difficult stage but exactly how it will impact their lives in future is just another of our constant concerns.

What was really disappointing was that many of the adults in our lives – some of them our closest friends and family – seemed totally overwhelmed by the diagnosis and the altered course of our lives. Perhaps they found themselves unable to cope. Or maybe we were the ones who'd changed. Whatever it was, many of them pulled away and, as a result, we often felt isolated and alone.

Throughout this time, Ian had been undergoing various blood tests and scans. We had been trying to remain positive but it was soon clear that Ian's PSA level had not decreased significantly enough. The recommendation now was for a course of salvage radiotherapy to be completed. So, once again, we faced a treatment decision.

The big sticking point here was that radiotherapy was something that Ian had firmly ruled out. He had watched his mum, dad and sis all undergo countless sessions and then suffer the consequences of further damage the treatment had caused. And, despite it all, they had still lost their battles.

But in Ian's case there was really no other option. It needed to be done. Once again, by scouring several websites I soon learned that there were many others around the world going through similar experiences. This knowledge filled us both with much-needed reassurance. It also revealed that there were many different options when it came to radiotherapy. So together this time, we developed a whole new list of questions to help keep us on track and ultimately make our decision.

After more research, we discovered one of our preferred oncologists consulted in a large public hospital, only about an hour from our home. This also meant we wouldn't have any out of pocket expenses for the treatment. We had heard great things about the entire team and were keen to get on their list but, of course, there was a long queue ahead of us.

One of the first challenges we faced in this new world was that time often stood still. In our previously active lives, we were not prepared for the endless waiting – waiting for test results, waiting for specialists, waiting for our life to begin again. It was like being broken down on the side of the highway watching the traffic flash past.

After eight weeks of daily radiotherapy each morning and trying to fit in a full day's work, we were both exhausted. This was the most difficult time. The stresses of a daily peak-hour commute, combined with waiting in a roomful of cancer patients while keeping the business going, was both physically draining and mentally exhausting. We were trying to be sympathetic to each other but it sure was tough going. It seemed one of us always needed to be stronger than the other. We took it in turns to fall apart and let the other pick up the slack.

We've both since been treated for depression and have also attempted to make some lifestyle changes to reduce stress and take a break. We've both found that meditation has helped and also that it's become increasingly important to have separate pastimes. This not only relieves tension but also provides much needed space apart from one another.

For me, it's been rediscovering the joys of writing and making it a commitment. For Ian, it has been finally allowing himself to take some *me-time*. To slow down and experience all the things he's always enjoyed: boating, fishing and travelling instead of always working.

Also, we've both become actively involved with prostate cancer support groups. We really felt that there was a need for more information to be made available to younger men and their partners. These men are in a totally different life stage to the usual demographic and are faced with many and varied issues. Just talking to someone closer to our age who has been through it all was exactly what we had needed. We both wanted to offer our experience to others.

Ian's treatments still have not reduced his PSA level sufficiently and, just as he had feared, it has increased many of the other problems he now endures on a daily basis. He's been back under the knife quite a few times and each time we hold our breath for bad news. So far, so good. But the unseen battle goes on, from bowel problems and bladder tumours to blood clots and nerve pain, plus increasing levels of tiredness and irritability, not to mention our old pals, incontinence and impotence. So the effects of the surgery and radiation are ongoing.

These days we're living from test to test waiting for the next result. We constantly have to remind ourselves that we're lucky – we've still got each other.

Meanwhile, we're stuck on this train. It's taking us up and over a steep, winding track down through deep, dark tunnels and out into vast barren fields. We still don't know where we're going but we know now that wherever it is, we'll reach our destination together.

Eclipse

Penny Gibson

Events crept up on us,
shadow by shadow.
PSA test. Diagnosis.
The world became silent,
expectant.

Look away, look elsewhere –
statistics, research.

Shadow measured by treatments:
radiotherapy, brachytherapy,
chemical orchiectomy.

Look away, look elsewhere –
Birdsville, Cape York.

Four fifths of the
promised time
vanished,
then pain, black blots
on the white shining bones.

Look away, look elsewhere –
lesions, catheters, urinary tract infections.

Chemotherapy, prednisolone,
taxotere, denosumab.
The penumbra insisted
until darkness was complete.
Endless pain-filled panic-filling nights.

Look away, look elsewhere –
morphine, sedation.

Zytiga ringed the black with promise.
The shadow was suspended.
Now, there's nowhere else to look,
nothing else to see
but the burning truth.

A Journey Through Cancer and Depression

Colin Bartlett

I experienced two symptoms that indicated the possibility of prostate cancer: blood in my urine and painful ejaculations. Knowing nothing about prostate cancer, I failed to immediately report my symptoms to my GP. When I finally did, my GP scheduled a blood test. I was 62, and as of this time a PSA test had not been initiated. Within four days there was a result with a PSA of 20. Consequently, my GP referred me to a urologist.

The urologist performed a DRE. Within seven days, I had a biopsy and a bone scan. The biopsy revealed a Gleason score of seven and the bone scan was clear. It was now one year since blood had appeared in my urine.

The urologist presented us with the diagnosis that I had an advanced case of prostate cancer and recommended an immediate prostatectomy; I had gone beyond the point of any choice.

My wife Trish and I left the urologist feeling hollow. What were we to do?

The word *cancer* spelt death to us.

A search for assistance on the web found the then-growing PCFA, who directed me to a PCA Support Group, Westmead.

With only one month from detection to a radical prostatectomy, information provided by members of The Westmead Prostate

Cancer Support Group filled in the gaps left by the GP and the urologist. We had made the correct choice, but lacked knowledge of pelvic floor exercises, something I had never done. This we now know is the key to a reasonably quick recovery from surgery.

I knew nothing about incontinence but soon realised it was affecting me and spent the next nine months calculating the urine leakage by weighing my incontinence pads on a set of kitchen scales, for want of a better method, to plot the progress of my recovery – a great therapy to remove one's mind from the 'real thing'.

The support group were excellent in their recommendations of what to do and, with their encouragement, I was back into an active life within a matter of weeks. Being a *keep-fit person*, I was back on my bike nine weeks after the radical.

Cancer makes people very self-centred. While I was moderately continent, I was suffering total erectional dysfunction. This, after many efforts, turned out to be total sexual dysfunction, such that you really do not feel concerned about your partner's problems. This was my lot!

Meanwhile Trish, my loving carer, was running around looking after me, making sure I was able to keep our business going. Poor Trish, whatever her feelings were, I didn't bother to ask; as long as I had my pads and my washing was done I was happy. She was the last on my list. It was a man thing!

The Westmead PCSG became an outlet and this led to me becoming a co-convenor. They proved to be a great way of sharing problems with others, although they were more oriented towards the male problems.

What is important here is the message I am trying to highlight: it was all about *me*!

Just over three years after the procedure, what next happened should have woken me to the problem of depression. I extended the morning exercise routine, going off for two to three hour bike rides. It was the only way I felt I could hide from my sexual frustration and the mental pain. Because nothing was happening, riding off into the sunrise and becoming involved with God's world was my way of staying on top of things. Worse was yet to come in this self-centred journey.

Incontinence returned, very badly. I could not mow the lawn without getting wet feet - and that was not from the grass. Getting up a ladder was not on and coughing or sneezing produced depressing results. It's all right if you wear dark pants, all you get is a warm feeling and nobody notices. If you don't mind, it doesn't matter, or does it?

We soldiered on for almost another three years when a series of events burst the cycle. My mother passed away suddenly. I had to go to the UK to settle her affairs; I came home distressed. Then followed three major seizures and a broken femur - trouble in large lumps, for Trish. She had to care for this wreck of a man.

With great help from a team of people - my GP, endocrinologist, neurologist and cardiologist - I ended up with a pacemaker as the seizures were due to an abnormally low heart rate, my general health being excellent. Yet, in all this, not one of them detected anything to do with depression.

Faith and trust play a big part in our recovery from the sadness and resultant depression created by prostate cancer and our ongoing health.

I sat at home for six months with Trish at my beck and call and became violent - not self-harm, just violent words and locking myself in a room. All I wanted to do was hide from this black hole that enveloped me, angry that I could not feel normal.

Poor Trish was frightened, called an ambulance and we ended up with two police cars and four policemen as well as two paramedics in the driveway.

This was the end. Trish broke down and I had to take her to our GP for help.

At this stage there had been a drive from Beyond Blue to educate not only PCSGs but also the GPs. I had ignored Beyond Blue up until this stage. However, our GP ran us both through their programme.

This was the first time I had heard of my depression; I was completely in denial. It was not me; it was everybody around me causing problems. That is the real self-centredness of depression.

The GP explained that my depression could be treated, which would assist Trish with her depression.

The effect of depression was far worse than the prostate cancer. So how did we stay rational in this period of time?

We are friends. After fifty-seven years together and fifty-five of them married, we are friends.

In our walk with the Lord we had spent up to two hours every day talking, discussing life and, above all, other people's problems.

Outside activities for me included Westmead PCSG, an Ambassador and Keynote Speaker for PCFA – this kept what balance there was on an even keel. It was my outburst that broke the situation and going to our GP for an explanation why.

GPs, together with the Beyond Blue programme, now have a great tool to assess patients with problems, then recommend them on for further treatment.

We both went onto a serotonin-enhancing medication and very quickly calmed down and started to enjoy life together again.

For Trish it gave her back the man that was hers!

For me it was a double cure. The medication also fixed my incontinence problem.

I asked Beyond Blue why this had happened. Their comment was that I was not thinking about it and all I had was 'stress incontinence'.

We learned from four physiotherapists that this medication is given in cases of angry bladder problems. It calms the bladder so the differential pressure between pelvic floor and bladder can become such that the sphincter in the pelvic floor can handle the changes in differential pressure.

So the key to recovery from depression and incontinence commences at the GP. They are the ones who can refer you to the correct clinician. They are the ones who can prescribe your medication. Your GP knows more about you than you do. Trust them. They are our lifeline to a happy and healthy lifestyle.

Recovery is very much in our Father's hands. The faith and trust He generates in us gives us the same faith and trust in our helpers. We still have anxious moments – only when too many problems fall on our plate. Ongoing medication has thankfully maintained a return to our previous love of life.

A Carer's Journey Through Clinical Depression

Trish Bartlett

When we were told that Colin had advanced prostate cancer and needed an operation straight away we were numb and shocked. We did not realise what a prostrate was or its function, but we wanted it out ASAP so we could get on with our lives.

The prostatectomy operation went well and we had the prospects of a good recovery. All the cancer had been caught, but we had concerns about incontinence and sexual dysfunction. Many members of our support group – the Westmead Prostate Cancer Support Group – appeared to have similar problems and we were optimistic that most of the problems would be overcome in time, especially with the encouragement of our support group members who were great.

Despite incontinence problems, Colin was able to get back to his fitness routine. Mentally and physically it was good for him. We were happy and accepted our lot. We knew things had changed. Always so close as a couple sexually, we missed that comfort due to our frustrating plumbing problems. It is not very nice to suddenly realise that your life partner is sick. You then are supposed to be understanding as a carer because you are not sick and your partner needs your support.

The journey into depression was not a conscious product of my responsibilities. It just grew on me. The anxiety I had became almost a normal day-to-day routine.

Having been together through the normal traumas associated with a failing business venture, this new challenge was somewhat camouflaged. Stress can easily creep in and wear you down. If an end is in sight you have something to pin your hopes to. Feelings of resentment and frustration for that person who has cramped your style can develop, especially if they are suffering with stress over what is happening to them and making things worse for you.

My beautiful man, my partner and friend of over 50-odd years was becoming someone I did not know. My strength was slowly running out.

Then to cap it all, to wake up in the night and find your beloved beside you having a major seizure created further panic and left me completely numb.

He was almost as good as dead. The paramedics came, assessed his condition as critical and took me, in my nightwear, to hospital with him. I had no thoughts of where I was going or how I was going to get home.

After seeming to settle down in hospital, Colin had another seizure and I thought this was it. He survived thanks to wonderful doctors and their skills. On getting Colin home he was no longer able to drive. I had to take him everywhere he had to go. He was a great backseat driver. I knew Colin was becoming more unwell but it was a chance comment by him, on my driving skills, that caused me to completely shut down. I felt I could no longer cope with his changing moods and his moments of anger.

I had such pain and fear taking care of him. It was only my husband – not a monster, but it seemed that at times a demon came into his mind. In now what seemed a desperate condition, Colin and I went to our GP – and friend – for some counselling.

He ran us both through the Beyond Blue programme to ascertain our situation with regards to depression. Following diagnosis as both being clinically depressed we were placed on a programme of antidepressants. The recovery was slow as we were both physically and mentally burnt out.

The medication, coupled with the Beyond Blue literature and our open discussions, brought us back to normality without any further counselling. Life is still great. It is wonderful to see the light at the end of the tunnel and find joy back in our lives. Depression can be destructive, but true love and our faith have created a relationship that is again as it was fifty-odd years ago.

Melancoyle Impostume

David Francis

'A canker is a melancolye impostume, eatynge partes
of the bodye.'

> – *Thomas Paynell (1528)*

A fleshy stone, a plum, resides beneath my bladder,
a crooked foetus, alive within its own time and space,
an unholy granite fixed within my gland.
Cell by cell it squeezes out its own specific antigen,
that grim excessive protein a signifier of things to come.
My tumour takes its long capricious walk
and creeps along tiny passages and larger carriageways
better used by semen and ejaculates.
It goes about my body, not thinking of conditions
or consequences, so set it is upon its fractured notion
of simply wanting more. It never sleeps.
This craggy rock is an avant-garde conception,
inept, a final metamorphosis withering my body,
blocking up my flow, facing down an awkward suicide.
Our elders thought disease was love transformed;
if so, this cull must be some crime of sickly passion,
or simply retribution for misplaced hungers of the past,
a melancolye impostume consuming to the end.

Waiting in Silence

Phillip McMillan

He doesn't seem worried, not even a little bit. Perhaps because he is the doctor and I am the patient. The test results show I don't have cancer, but his confidence and lack of concern does not make me feel any better, because for the first time in my life death is looking over my shoulder.

I don't have cancer, never did have cancer, and probably never will have cancer, but I know that the very essence of me, the atoms and molecules that built me into me, are not as they should be. They have mistakes. The very molecular programming in every cell, in every part of my body, has become a source of danger instead of a source of wonderment. Where prostate cancer is concerned, I chose bad DNA. My father, Norm, died of prostate cancer; my uncles have prostate cancer; my cousin died of prostate cancer; and now my brother has prostate cancer.

The first thing you learn as a Buddhist is that you will die. You will get old, get sick, and die. That is, if you are fortunate enough to have avoided the proverbial bus coming down the street or an unexpected heart attack while taking the dog for a walk. I have studied the theory and understand the doctrine that I should prepare for a good death. That's what Buddhists do: we know we will die so we prepare for it - to have a good death! But I'm only 48 years old and startled that I need to prepare so early. I wasn't expecting this; not now, not yet.

Prostate cancer sneaks up on you while you're having a glass of wine with friends. It doesn't come when you're a young risk-taker bungee jumping in New Zealand or riding a motorbike without a helmet in rural India. No! Prostate cancer comes at a time in your life when you seem to have it all together. Your career develops and you feel as though you are in the position to achieve great things; the kids grow up and start to earn their own money or, with a bit of luck, move out completely. For the first time, life doesn't seem as hard as it once was, and you actually enjoy having more time to spend with your wife. But, just as you are planning that trip to China to walk the Great Wall and see what is so forbidden about the Forbidden City, prostate cancer is inserted into the family conversation.

Back at the doctor's office, I surmise that I will need to change my lifestyle, I will need to do all the right things to maximise my chances – I might even have to cut down my drinking. So I start to ask questions about my lifestyle and what I can do to reduce my chances of developing cancer. The doctor says the number one thing to do is to stop smoking, but I don't smoke; I have not had a cigarette for 30 years. What about diet? Well, apart from maintaining a normal healthy diet and a normal weight, there is not really much diet will do. It's not just a matter of eating more brussels sprouts.

The doctor thinks for a minute.

I like this – that's what I'm paying him for. *Get those brain cells working, Doc!* After a suitable gathering of thoughts, he is ready to impart the wisdom learned from years of training and experience.

'There is one thing we can do that we know will stop you getting prostate cancer.'

I lean forward in my seat. 'Yes, yes, go on.'

'We could cut your balls off.'

A stabbing chill moves slowly down my body. It starts in my ears as the words strike my cochlea and inner ear, then moves through my face, down my neck and circles my heart three times before punching me in the stomach and sinking lower to my testicles. I look like a kangaroo caught in the headlights of a car. He could have cut my balls off right there and then and I would have been powerless to stop him.

It seems like a long time, but in reality must have only been a few seconds.

'Mmm, I didn't think you would go for that,' he says with a wry smile. 'Don't worry about your cousin; he's too far away in the family tree. Yes, your dad had cancer, but he was much older than you. Most cancers are very slow-growing, and men die of old age while waiting for the cancer to grow. Okay, now, your brother – that is a concern, because he's only 51 and his is fast-growing. But his doctor caught it very early and I'm sure he will be just fine. The important thing is regular testing. You need to have a blood test and physical examination every year. Apart from that, go home, have a glass of wine, make love to your wife and don't worry.' He repeats in an authoritative tone, 'You don't have cancer and may never have cancer.'

I go home and follow the doctor's advice – he is a doctor, after all.

But life has changed. It has become a lot more serious. Dad was one of six children: three boys and three girls. Over the last few years, there have been numerous family funerals – Mum and Dad's generation have started to pass away. It must have been hard for Mum to see her family and friends die, to go to funerals like she once went to weddings. I go when I can and it's always sad to see them go, but it is never threatening because they are not my generation; they are expected to go first, that's the natural order of things. But now my generation is getting sick, my generation is dying. My cousin, whom I grew up with, is dead and my brother is sick, and I'm worried by the fact that there is very little I can do to improve my situation without having my balls cut off.

The whole story started in 1997 when my father, Norm, was diagnosed with prostate cancer. We took it very seriously, because just two years earlier we had watched Ted Whitten waving a sad goodbye to sports fans while being driven for the last time around the MCG. If prostate cancer could do that to a goliath like Ted, then imagine what it could do to a mere mortal like Dad.

Dad was about 63 at the time and had been retired for about eight years after a life working in the railways. He was a quiet man who enjoyed the quiet things in life, like a glass of cold beer, watching the football on TV, and fishing on the beach at Noosa every winter. He was very close to Mum and didn't like to be separated from her; it had always been that way. He was a good bloke, but I struggled to get to know him as a man.

I knew him as a father – and a good father he was. As kids, we would jump all over him in the backyard and he would fight us off with rough play that young boys thrive on. We would line up to take turns receiving a back scratch from him by the fire on a cold winter's night. He would cook barbeques and take us camping at Rosebud on the Mornington Peninsula. We spent nights at the carnival and days at the beach. We never wanted for anything; we weren't rich, but we weren't poor. I had a happy childhood, but as I grew older and had my own children, I wanted to get to know my father more – not as a father, but as a man.

But Dad was a hard man to get to know; he just didn't open up and talk about the dreams and disappointments of his life. His generation put up with most hardships because they didn't expect things to go well anyway. They expected more problems in life than my generation does, and standard procedure was to say nothing and just get on with it. Get up each morning at 5.30 am and catch the train to work, even if you no longer find it very stimulating – it wasn't called work for nothing, you know!

When Dad had the opportunity to take an early retirement, he grabbed it with both hands; getting paid not to come to work seemed like a dream come true. But he didn't have a plan; free from the burden of earning a paycheque, he struggled to know how to fill in the time. There just didn't seem to be anything he was longing to do – no bucket list, no hobby, no diversion from sitting in the chair reading the newspaper. I tried all sorts of approaches to get him active and involved so that we could spend more time together. I tried buying him golf clubs so we could play golf together, but it was not really his thing. I tried inviting him to the football, but no, he would rather stay at home with Mum. It was a one-way street; I was trying and he wasn't.

Then, for no reason at all, Dad's brother Ron developed prostate cancer. Dad figured he had better get a check-up and the resulting blood tests showed high readings; Dad also had prostate cancer. Why? Nobody could say. There was nothing to be done but to accept the situation and follow the medical advice. As you would expect, this put a dampener on the whole situation, and a close relationship with my father became even harder. Not strained, because there was no tension, no fights, no drama, but the task of getting to know my father as a man was now moving beyond reach. Conversations with Mum became about the treatment and Dad withdrew even further. He was still there and we could talk about football, politics and other superficial things, but we could not talk about us, about him, about me. Two men having a quiet beer became two men having a quiet beer.

As expected, most prostate cancers are slow to grow, so while there was concern, a lot more tests needed to be done to see how much of a concern there was. A biopsy revealed cancer in about 50% of the samples taken. Radiation was advised and that was the course of action taken. Dad had a great sense of duty and he never made a fuss or complained too much over the months of radiation, but he was not well at all.

Dad was hardly eating and it looked like his body had started to shrink; visits and conversations were punctuated with long silences. What could I talk to him about? What could I do to put a smile on his face? Talking about the treatment did nothing for the situation at all, and it was pointless asking him anyway, as he knew and I knew that Mum gave me all this information anyway. If only I could find one thing that he was really passionate about, that one thing that excited him, maybe I could have made this an easier time for him and a special time for the both of us. In many ways I felt a failure because, after studying him for more than 40 years, I felt I had only been allowed to scratch the surface of his personality and what gave him joy.

But maybe I was trying to impose my expectations of him on him. He was probably just happy watching his children grow up and raise their own families. Maybe he didn't need to be involved – maybe he was happy just being quietly proud. In all likelihood it was my problem and not his. But watching him suffer, watching him deteriorate and not being able to fix the problem or being able to help in a way that would bring us closer together, was tough. I knew that once time was gone, it would be lost forever. The time would be gone but the loss would stay. It was something I had to keep to myself too; had I made a fuss, I would have looked like a spoilt child craving attention while my father was fighting for his life.

The treatment and silence worked and the cancer went into remission. Mum and Dad seemed to have a new spring in their step and jumped straight in the car and headed for Queensland. Dad liked fishing on the beach, a silent personal occupation that suited him well. They got to know other couples up there that were the same age and looked forward to the three-month trip every winter.

Mum would send an occasional email but Dad avoided the computer, so all communication was through Mum and even then it was sparse. My family have never been great at communicating, not then and not now. Even me; sometimes it's easier to put words on a page than it is to discuss things with the family. But the reality is that those five years of remission were probably the retirement Dad was looking for, the one he had always wanted.

During this time, news was filtering through that Dad's other brother, Len, also had prostate cancer. That's three out of three brothers with the same disease! It looked more than a coincidence. I was just over 40 and attention started to be drawn onto my generation. There were eleven males in my generation from the six

McMillan siblings on my father's side; I was the fourth youngest. We started to request checks from our doctors and most of us started yearly blood and physical examinations. We were now on the lookout for it. My doctor wasn't concerned at all. There was no reason at all to think that I was at risk at 42.

But for the first time in my life, my health was an active concern.

Dad, Ron and Len all seemed to battle though with radiation and various forms of treatment and all went into remission. Tough guys, those McMillan men; they all showed strength that I had never given them credit for.

After about five years in remission, Dad was having one of his check-ups; he had all but forgotten about the cancer. But it had not forgotten about him. Results showed alarmingly high levels in the blood and a physical examination revealed a rough surface on the prostate. It was back, and this time it was serious. The cancer had a newfound vigour and hostility. The medical team had real concerns that it had already started to spread. Removing the prostate may well have been a painful, dangerous and useless exercise. A series of patches and skin implants were started; these were kept up for three months but didn't really seem to be doing much, so his treatment was upgraded to chemo.

The chemo was very tough on Dad, but he had beaten the cancer once and he showed confidence that he could do it again. I had been waiting a long time to see this. He was angry. How dare this bloody thing come back for seconds! I had waited 20 years of my adult life to see this outbreak of emotion, and it made me feel proud. I didn't tell him that, but I was really proud of the outrage and it made me feel closer to him, even if I never said it. I always felt that, if I did say something, it would have been interpreted as me saying that last goodbye because the men in my family never did talk. To all of a sudden start now may even be discouraging.

For all the fight and all the medical intervention, he didn't have much success this time around. About four months into the contest, those around him knew that he would not stand on the dais for this one.

In parallel to watching my father rapidly decline, our beloved family dog Casey was 18 years old, blind and senile with no quality of life. He was a little white long-haired Chihuahua – my wife Joanne's dog, really – but he had been there every moment with my two daughters as they grew up. Dogs are always there for you; dogs show love and emotion every time you see them. People don't, but dogs do.

I would see Casey every day and hope that he could die peacefully in his sleep, knowing that we should make the decision ourselves and not leave it to fate. It was a big moral quandary and it troubled me greatly. Somehow, my mind had set itself up so that to euthanise Casey was to give up on my father. I just could not do it.

Dad spent about another five months in and out of hospital until the day came when we knew that this was to be his final admittance. He would not come home this time. Various members of the family would visit every day and do our best to talk, not just to a quiet man, but a quiet man who was dying. He was overly concerned about silly things like the possibility that he could no longer drive a car. This really did seem to concern him, but I knew he would not come home from hospital, let alone drive a car. As the time got closer, we knew the final moment would be soon. Mum, Mum's sister Rosemary, brother Gary, sister Andrea and I all gathered in the palliative care section to help him make the journey. Dad had his own timetable and kept us up all night without any change. The next afternoon, while I was at work, word came through that Dad was gone; Mum and Rosemary had been there for him every minute so, thankfully, he didn't die alone. I went to the hospital but didn't really know what to do. There was nothing to do. The quiet man had gone quietly.

Being the first of the six siblings to pass away, Dad's funeral was a big affair, and I was called upon for the main eulogy. A complicated task at any time, but how could I do the man justice and do my duty when the reality was that I had struggled to know him? In Dad's final week, I tossed and turned every night working through draft speeches in my mind. There are no second chances here. You only get one chance to do it right. But what is right? I resolved that he should be asked if he wanted to say anything. I knew I should ask him, that he should be given the opportunity, but how? How do you discuss funeral arrangements with a dying man when you have struggled to talk for the last twenty years? It had to be done, so in a private moment I asked.

'When the time comes, whenever that is, is there anything you want me to say?'

He looked directly at me. 'You will know what to say,' his soft voice came back to me. His eyes did all the talking, really.

He had faith in me. After more than forty years, he had faith in me.

When the time came and the people of his life were assembled, I performed my duty, just like he had all his life. I did the eulogy and I did a good one at that. I felt that it was the one thing I had control over, the one thing I could do. It felt good.

Two weeks after Dad died, I sat in the lounge room and held Casey. I cried and cried. I told Joanne it was time but that I could not do it. She would have to take him to the vet by herself.

Dad died in 2004, and with Ron and Len also having prostate cancer, my brother Gary and I were getting yearly checks, both blood tests and physical exams. We knew we were at risk but also that we were young and there was no need for concern. My doctor certainly was not concerned.

Around this time, I was travelling a lot for business. I would do about eight or ten overseas trips a year to places like India, Bangladesh, China, Sri Lanka and Thailand. A little bit of overseas business travel is great, but a lot can actually become a burden, and it seemed that when I would travel something would always go wrong back home. In 2006, both Steve Irwin and Peter Brock unexpectedly died in tragic circumstances. Paul Newman, Heath Ledger, Pavarotti, Evel Knievel and Michael Jackson all made the supreme sacrifice while I sat alone in a three-star hotel room somewhere in Asia; for a moment there I felt that each time I would travel, a celebrity had to die.

In 2010, I was in India sitting in my hotel room by myself and on the shaky hotel internet connection, when I got an email from my mother saying my cousin, Michael, had prostate cancer. It had moved on to the next generation, to Michael, who was the eldest of my cousins, whom I grew up with and went to the swimming club with as a child. He was the first in the family to go to university, he had done well in life, and everyone liked Michael. Most prostate cancers are slow-growing, but not Michael's. His was an aggressive bastard, a heavyweight fighter intent on bullying and beating up an ordinary guy.

The word through the family grapevine was that nobody was sure how this would turn out. All this came at a time when he was at the peak of his life. Things were really good; he had a happy marriage, a great career, and a lovely granddaughter. His passion was France and he and his wife would travel every year to the French countryside to drink wine with friends. Life was better than ever, and at that moment he was chosen to get terminal cancer. It had no regard for what the man had to offer society. In the end, he didn't really stand a chance; it devoured him like it ultimately devoured Dad the second time around.

When Michael was sick, I wanted to see him, to comfort him – just to talk, really, but I never did. It was complicated. While he was my cousin and we grew up around the corner from each other, we didn't really see each other on a regular basis. You leave school and develop a new circle of friends away from your family. People tend to drift apart. We would see each other on family occasions and would chat and enjoy each other's company on such occasions, but it was not a regular thing. For me to all of a sudden turn up and want to chat when he was terminally ill would be to drive a nail in the man's coffin. Turning up to say a last goodbye might have made me feel good, but I could not see anything in it for him.

I had to watch from afar, watch and wait, wait and watch. Emails would come through giving various glimpses of hope, but I knew Michael would not make it. I was torn in my soul. Michael had affected me greatly, even more than Dad had, but surely this was a selfish attitude? Oh, sure, I cared about Michael because he was just four years older than me. I could see this was not the person I wanted to be. It upset me greatly to be so self-centred.

But I am now in the same situation as Michael before his cancer. It's a carbon copy. Life is great and things are going really well. Life is less of a struggle than it was when the kids were young and housing interest rates were 18%. The mortgage is no longer a problem and I don't need to make home brew anymore because I can afford to buy real beer. My daughters are doing just fine; both are engaged and are building careers and lives for themselves. After 20 years of raising children, the time has come for my wife Joanne and I to have some 'us' time. But there are no guarantees. I know that. I am a Buddhist, after all. I understand the law of impermanence. Things will always change.

They sure did change for Michael, but am I next?

When Michael died, it was a shock. We knew it would happen, but it was still a shock. A shock of disbelief that a good man in his prime could be cut down so abruptly. We didn't want to believe it, but there we were, in the same funeral chapel that had hosted Dad's funeral, listening to a eulogy just like the one I had given for Dad a few years earlier. I cried, sitting in the chapel, I cried; I didn't cry at Dad's funeral but I did this time.

My brother Gary wasn't at Michael's funeral; he was in hospital. Two weeks before, his doctor had detected a slight rise in his PSA, a rise that under normal circumstances would just trigger a wait-and-see approach. A physical exam was inconclusive, but a rough patch on the prostate was detected. His General Practitioner was very cautious and did not want to take risks, so she sent him to a specialist who wanted a biopsy. Gary was getting a biopsy while we were at Michael's funeral; the whole situation seemed surreal.

During the next week, I held back and waited to get word about Gary's condition from Mum rather than look like I was conducting a watch on my brother. I always thought it would look selfish of me to make too much of a fuss. Gary and I had never spent a lot of time together as adults. As kids, I was the younger brother who had always wanted to do what he was doing.

'Why can't I go too?' and 'He's got one, I want one' and 'That's not fair.'

I was the pain-in-the-arse little brother, and when he left home he didn't see the need to have his little brother still hanging around. It was my fault, not his, but it all meant that as adults we had never been close. To suddenly develop overt attention to my brother seemed fake, even if it was real, even if it was out of genuine compassion.

All this is what happens when men don't talk. We fill in the blanks to missing spots in conversations that we never actually had. Conversations that only occurred in our mind because we didn't quite know how to start the dialogue. We weren't scared to talk – we just didn't know how.

Gary had cancer! There was cancer in two of the eighteen samples. The medical team had got to the disease very early, and the chances of it having already spread were low. He was 51 and he didn't have death looking over his shoulder anymore; it was staring at him, right in the eyes, like a violent drunk in a suburban nightclub. As we know, prostate cancer comes in two types: aggressive and slow. Gary had the same aggressive type that killed Michael; another 12 months unchecked and Gary would have been paying a close personal visit to Michael. But they did catch it in time and his prognosis was good. We always felt confident Gary could beat it. The silence and distance was more than I could handle, so I started to call around to his home or ring to see how he was going.

Do you know what happens when you break the silence? When someone makes a first move? When someone asks, 'How are you?'

People talk, that's what happens – even with men it can happen. Men can talk, men can show compassion, and men can accept and appreciate that they have others around them who care for them and who are fighting with them.

We started to see each other more while Gary was evaluating treatment options. He was told to lose ten kilograms and get fit, get ready for a fight. Which is exactly what he did; he fought like a prize-fighter, and I was proud. He was a determined man, determination I had never seen before. Maybe it was there all along and I just wasn't there to see it, but I saw it now. We discussed the pros and cons of each available option, openly and honestly. These are not easy decisions to make and there is no simple path to take. Each treatment has different probabilities and each treatment has its own list of side effects. That one crisp clear standout perfect solution doesn't exist. Whichever way is chosen, it's a compromise.

Gary opted for full removal of the prostate because the cancer was so fast-growing and they had caught it so early. It was his best chance to beat the disease once and for all, the best chance for long-term survival. He had a great surgeon and after the operation, all tests showed him to be cancer-free.

So the story comes back to me. Gary's surgeon suggested that I get checked every six months rather than every year. This seemed sensible to me. I could not see any downside to getting checked more often. My best chance was frequent testing. That way, if I did get cancer, we should get to it early and I should be okay.

So now I wait ...

You can't live on high alert all the time, and even if you could, it would defeat the whole purpose. Imagine that you could find out exactly when, where, and how you would die. Would you want to know? Every night, my mind plays through a thousand scenarios of my demise. This must be how the CIA work playing spy games. I started to work on the songs for my funeral and made a special playlist on my iPod.

> 'Knocking on Heaven's Door' – Bob Dylan
> 'Seasons in the Sun' – Terry Jacks
> 'The Nips are Getting Bigger' – Mental as Anything
> 'Wonderful World' – Louis Armstrong
> 'My Sweet Lord' – George Harrison
> 'Up Around the Bend' – Credence Clearwater Revival

I listen to these songs over and over again. Instead of making me sad and depressed about my possible doom, they make me happy; they remind me how great life is. It's a cliché to say that a near-death experience – or, in my case, a realisation that I am high-risk – makes you re-evaluate your life. But all clichés have an element of truth to them, and I had been re-evaluating my life for some time anyway.

I went back to the man who had served me well for advice in the past, His Holiness the Dalai Lama, and I came up with a radical theory to life.

I would say 'yes' instead of saying 'no'.

It was so simple – that was the beauty of it. Stop hesitating. Stop saying 'I'm too busy' and say 'yes' to new experiences. Join Rotary? Okay. Go scuba diving? Okay. Write a book? Why not? I really don't have time to get cancer. It's not about the waiting anymore. I certainly don't feel the need to get my balls cut off.

When you start saying yes to things instead of saying no, life gets better. You open your mind to new experiences. Maybe you really do like spicy food, maybe the ballet is a good night's entertainment, after all. Have you ever been to Hong Kong? Why not? What's holding you back? What are you waiting for? Cancer?

It's not quite the concept of a bucket list; it's a bit more like not wanting to waste time. The Dalai Lama has a saying: 'Enlightenment; if not now, when?' It pretty well sums up my position nowadays.

I am now happier and more content than I ever have been in my life, I don't know what the future holds, but I don't intend to dwell on it and don't really want to know. All the new experiences I have build me into a better me, a better husband, a better father and a better community member than I was before.

It's not that my life completely changed because of my family experience with prostate cancer, but it goes into the mix of my life experiences that have shaped my attitudes and made me who I am today. I have started to communicate a lot better with the people around me; I see my brother much more often and I'm not scared to talk about problems. That male cone of silence is breaking down. It's still there, but it is diminishing.

When my time comes, I will have no regrets. Be it in one year or in forty years, I will know I did the best I could. So I get tested every six months, drink wine, make love, travel, help the community where I can and watch my daughters grow into healthy, strong, independent women with good hearts.

Life is good.

How Archery Helped Me Get Through Prostate Cancer

Dermot McKeone

I wasn't sure whether to start this story with the prostate cancer or the archery. As I started shooting arrows before I discovered my prostate problem, I'd better start with the archery.

I retired in 2007 at the age of 62 and my wife thought I ought to do something apart from growing vegetables and writing my blog. I didn't think I needed another pastime, but as she'd given me a voucher for a four-week archery course for my 63rd birthday, I thought I'd better give it a try, though it took me six months before I got round to using the voucher.

So at the end of September 2008, I started my course with AC Delco Bowmen in Eastleigh. I didn't do too badly in the first lesson, and by the time I was through that initial two-hour session, I'd decided that I'd carry on with the sport after the course. Within weeks, I'd bought my own recurvebow; by Christmas I was shooting indoors with the club at a local school; by February the following year I was totally hooked.

The summer of 2009 passed in a haze. In May, I won a novice's competition at 60, 50 and 40 yards; later that summer I migrated to longer distances, and started working towards a classification. I ended the year a 2nd Class Archer.

Like so many older guys who don't bother too much about their health, I discovered my prostate problem accidentally. In the autumn of that year, I'd been talking to my doctor about the discomfort I'd been having after driving, and, in my ignorance, suggested that there might be a prostate problem causing it.

It wasn't (it was a minor hernia) but he did say that we might as well check my PSA as I'd mentioned it.

'Yes, by all means, let's do it,' I said cheerfully. I was so not bothered.

A few days later the test results came back and I was a little concerned to hear that my PSA level was higher than it should be … and so commenced a winter of tests and hospital visits that culminated with my operation on 30 June 2010.

The evening after I had my biopsy I was due to shoot indoors at the club. I asked the doctor who took the sample if I'd be okay to shoot some arrows that night. He said he felt it would be fine. I shot appallingly that night, on two occasions missing the target completely. Whether it was my state of mind or the massive dose of antibiotics following the biopsy that caused this I'm not sure, but I decided to go home after about a dozen ill-directed arrows.

The biopsy results weren't encouraging, and after a confirmatory MRI scan, I opted for radical prostatectomy using keyhole surgery.

Apart from the night after the biopsy, my archery performance was surprisingly unaffected. A few weeks before my op, I shot my first 1st Class score and I was shooting right up until the weekend I went into hospital. I asked my surgeon how long it would be before I could start shooting again afterwards; much to my surprise, he suggested that about three weeks would probably be enough, but I should wait until afterwards to see how I felt.

Keyhole surgery is amazing. Although I felt pretty ropey for ten days or so after the op, thanks to having to use a catheter, I was bouncing around like a teenager after they removed it. Two weeks after the op I was coping well and went for a three-mile walk. A week later, as forecast, I was ready to get back to my sport. I'd lost very little muscle tone during the weeks and I pretty much carried on where I had left off. I guess it was down to the fact that archery is very much a mental and upper-body-strength sport.

During the weeks of my continuing recovery over that summer and autumn, archery provided a focus and a distraction. My scores continued to improve and I ended the year a 1st Class Archer. I maintained this for two years. I haven't quite maintained this standard since then, and I doubt now whether I'll progress to the next level – 'Bowman'. As my knowledge and technical ability improves, my body is getting older and I think the two trends are counteracting one another. One bit of my body, however, is no longer a cause for concern, and my PSA level was back down to zero last time I checked.

In 2011, I became an archery coach. I have coached a number of older men and I would be delighted to talk to any potential archers travelling the prostate journey, perhaps going on one of our introductory courses.

I would advise any man going through the prostate procedure to keep up (or take up) a sport of some kind, whether it's something non-competitive like swimming, or something more intensive like archery or squash. Obviously, it's a good idea to check with your doctor before you take up anything too strenuous.

To summarise, here is what archery did for me over the period of my diagnosis, operation and recovery:

- archery took my mind off the tests and hospital visits
- it gave me something to aim for (literally!) while all this was going on
- it kept me fit – I was in pretty good nick when I had my operation
- I was able to take up my sport again pretty much straight after the operation
- it continues to give me good levels of exercise
- archery mostly uses the muscles of the upper body – the stuff going on downstairs doesn't get in the way too much!

And if you, the reader, are on this journey, I wish you the very best of luck - and who knows, maybe I'll see you on an archery range some time!

The Song of the Prostate Gland

Dermot Dorgan

Come all you good red-blooded men, I will not keep you long.
Just sit right there with your bum in the chair, 'cos you
need to hear this song.
It'll end and start with a body part that's famed
throughout the land
as a source of pride, but of grief beside, and it's called the
prostate gland.

And this is the song of the prostate gland; let's sing it long and loud,
'cos in the end it's a boy's best friend, may it always do you proud.

Now the prostate's not a glamour gland, unlike the brain
and the heart.
You'll find it lyin' where the sun don't shine on an
anatomical chart.
But the job it does gives us all a buzz, as we reach that
point ecstatic.
From the heights of Zeus, what is then produced is of
origin prostatic.

And this is the song of the prostate gland; let's sing it high and low,
in that circumstance, you may feel like Clancy of the (ahem) overflow.

But time goes by and the years just fly and your prostate
ages too,
and one fine day, you just may hear words that will shock
you through –
'You should be aware that there's cancer there.' And my
mind anticipates,
and in seconds flat it has me on the mat outside the
Pearly Gates.

And this is the song of the prostate gland; let's sing it to the end,
'cos if you miss hell's fire, there's the heavenly choir to drive you
'round the bend.

The doctor said, 'No, you're not dead – that's all just in
your mind.'
He went on to say there's a couple of ways, he could help
me out of my bind.
'We could whip it out, and there's little doubt you'd
avoid annihilation,
or we could cut the crap and give it a zap with nuclear radiation.'

And this is the song of the prostate gland; let's sing it like a lark,
but I was scared of the chance that my underpants would be
glowing in the dark.

Well, I was in some strife, so I chose the knife to get me
cancer-clear.
With events in Japan, I thought I'd put a ban on any
more radiation over here.
So they went ahead and I woke in bed, all stitched up
and sore,
with blood all about and a tube coming out where there
never was a tube before.

And this is the song of the prostate gland come sing along with me.
But the truth to tell was it hurt like hell to even have a pee.

Now I'm recovering fast and I've seen the last (I hope) of
the dreaded C.
And although that's nice, still you pay a price for being
cancer-free.
Your male prowess is a bit of a mess, 'til recovery comes again.
And you tend to leak like Breakfast Creek after weeks of
Brisbane rain.

And this is the song of the prostate gland; let's sing it high and low.
And if you've cash to spare, then Viagra shares might be the
way to go.

So come all you good red-blooded men, I wish you all the best.
Don't just stand with your head in the sand, but do the
prostate test.
If it comes out clear, you can give a cheer, and you won't
have to join the strugglers,
And you'll thank your stars that you show no scars when
you wear your budgie smugglers.

And this is the end of the prostate song. It's gone on far too long,
And if the test's adverse, and you fear the worst, you can always
sing this song.

Getting Along with Hormone Therapy

Peter Simpson

Recently I turned 71, which made me realise I've been living with prostate cancer for nine years. When first diagnosed I decided not to have a radical prostatectomy and instead finished up having three different kinds of treatment – brachytherapy, cryotherapy and hormone therapy. The brachytherapy kept the cancer suppressed and confined to the prostate for several years, but the cryotherapy only had a very temporary benefit. After that it was too late to consider surgical removal as those treatments had left me with too much damage around the prostate. The only option left was hormone therapy – something I'd being trying to avoid.

It has taken a long time to come to terms with the fact that I'm going to be on hormone therapy, along with all its dismal side effects, for the rest of my life, but I have learned to live with the situation and along the way I've found that some of these effects can be lessened or made a little easier to cope with.

Case History

In August 2004 my GP told me that I'd better have my prostate checked. My PSA had risen from 2.0 to 2.7 in the space of four months, and the GP recommended a visit to a specialist.

Sure enough, by an astonishingly quick and effective method, the urologist found a lump on my prostate and recommended a trans-rectal ultrasound-guided (TRUS) biopsy.

He explained to me that this initial finding (the lump) almost certainly meant early-stage prostate cancer rather than just an infection or some other minor trouble, but that any cancer at this stage would be confined to the prostate, not running riot through the rest of my body. It was therefore quite treatable and I wasn't going to die of cancer in the near future. I took him at his word, but still felt scared at the idea of having cancer at all, treatable or not. From what little I knew of the subject, cancer always turned out to be lethal, sooner or later. I broke the news to my wife Valerie that afternoon, and she was even more alarmed than I was.

The biopsy confirmed the presence of cancer in about 50% of the gland, with a Gleason score of six.

Radical Prostatectomy or Radiation Brachytherapy?
The next specialist was a radiation oncologist who thought I was an ideal candidate for brachytherapy. In later years I wondered if having brachytherapy was the right decision, but the radiation oncologist and his colleague – the surgeon-urologist – whose patient I had by then become, convinced me without too much persuasion that this was the best path to follow.

There was another reason why I chose brachytherapy rather than have the whole prostate surgically removed. A couple of years before, Valerie had been stricken with a rare and paralysing condition called Chronic Inflammatory Demyelinating Polyneuropathy (CIDP). At the time we were living in Tennant Creek in the Northern Territory, where I was a geologist looking for the next big goldmine and Valerie was training Aboriginal people to be school teachers. We both gave up these interesting and satisfying jobs and moved to Melbourne. Valerie then spent most of 2003 and 2004 in Royal Melbourne Hospital, including a total of 11 months in Intensive Care. It was amazing that she survived. It left her with a lot of damage, and I became her primary carer. She was mostly confined to a wheelchair and needed help with almost every aspect of daily living. On top of all this she had to use a ventilator all night to breathe – her sleep mechanism was compromised and although she could get through the whole day breathing for herself, she couldn't go fully to sleep and breathe for herself at the same time.

However, there was nothing wrong with her brain and the two of us adjusted to our new set of conditions quite well. I did the cooking, shopping, laundry, driving, paying the bills and all the general running around, as well as helping her with the many things involved in caring for a disabled person. Valerie's contributions lay in getting our apartment organised and furnished, keeping in contact with our family and friends, dealing with the support services (we had a Melbourne City Council carer come in most days to give Valerie her morning shower, a service for which I am profoundly grateful) and just being a happy and supportive companion. If that sounds like an uneven distribution of the work, it never seemed that way. We have now been living contentedly like this for eight years and it has been, perhaps surprisingly, a very happy time.

So, given Valerie's disability, there were limits to how long I felt I could leave her by herself on any given day and although there were a few other people around who could and sometimes did look after her well, I did not like the idea of leaving her alone, or in the care of others, for too long. That was a powerful reason why I was more inclined to have brachytherapy, which would only put me out of action for a couple of days, whereas having a radical prostatectomy would have left me unable to care for my wife for several weeks.

Brachytherapy

In November 2004 I had the brachytherapy operation at Freemasons Hospital. The radiation from the Iodine-125 'seeds' had a half-life of 60 days. Having been a geologist I just happened to have an old Geiger counter tucked away in a cupboard. If I held this antique gadget out at arm's length it would just tick away gently, but when I swung it in towards my groin the clicking would speed up until it reached a high-pitched squeal. I used to call this my 'party trick'. As the months went by the radiation faded away, as it was supposed to do, and I was no longer able to amuse or horrify people with my little demonstration.

The radiation treatment had a good and lasting effect. My PSA quickly dropped to around 0.5 and was satisfactorily steady at around that level for about four years, but eventually it began to rise again. About then, just to make life difficult, the defective heart valve I'd had from birth began to fail, so I had to undergo heart surgery to install an artificial aortic valve, a length of Dacron aorta and a pacemaker. From then on I needed daily doses of Warfarin.

In the year up to January 2009 my PSA level rose to 5.9. A biopsy confirmed the re-growth of the cancer. This time the Gleason score was seven. Scans found no tumours outside the prostate and it was assumed that the cancer was still encapsulated, but something had to be done and the options were limited.

Cryotherapy and Hormone Therapy
My urologist told me I would have to start hormone therapy, as I had reached my limit of radiation treatment. Radical prostatectomy was ruled out because the radiation and cryotherapy damage to the surrounding tissue might lead to a bladder-colon fistula, which would almost certainly mean having to wear a colostomy bag forevermore. High-Intensity Focused Ultrasound (HIFU) wouldn't work because the implanted 'seeds' would deflect the beams away from the target tumours. I'm not sure, but proton beam methods might not work either for the same reason and anyway, it wasn't available in Australia. I was very reluctant to have hormone therapy because of the castration effects and other bodily changes which I found rather frightening.

By this time I'd been doing a lot of hunting around on the internet to try and find an alternative to the recommended hormone therapy, and eventually sought a second opinion. I felt uncomfortable doing this – it was as though I was cheating on my regular urologist. But I went ahead and the second opinion man suggested I have 'salvage cryotherapy', which meant having the prostate spiked with carefully-placed needles in which super-cooled liquid argon was circulated, freezing the whole prostate solid and cracking up the cancer tumour molecules. Bladder and colon are filled with circulating warm water to try and keep the freezing confined to just the prostate. This technique was only carried out at St George Hospital in Sydney. My regular urologist hadn't known that this was available, so getting this second opinion proved quite justified.

I pinned a lot of hope on this cryotherapy idea, hoping it would kill off all the cancerous cells once and for all. I flew to Sydney, had an encouraging meeting with the surgeon and it was arranged that I would have the salvage cryotherapy done at the next opportunity.

Then followed a worrying period while I waited to hear when the cryotherapy might happen. It dragged on for a year and a half. The NSW hospital system seemed to be in disarray; cryotherapy wasn't regarded as a mainstream treatment (despite being done successfully for over 12 years) and funding had been withdrawn. The surgeon wasn't at all responsive to my phone and fax questions so after seven months had passed I flew to Sydney again for another face-to-face talk with him, but even this didn't produce a firm date.

It was risky to wait any longer while my PSA level kept rising rapidly, in case the cancer began to metastasise, so very reluctantly I started hormone therapy, in March 2009, while still waiting for the cryotherapy. Maybe the two therapies acting in tandem would produce the desired result. I had four of these Eligard (leuprolide acetate) injections, at four-monthly intervals. My PSA readings quickly went down and stayed at under 0.5.

NSW Government funding for cryotherapy was finally reinstated and eventually I had it done in August 2010. I was still hoping that it was going to rid me of prostate cancer totally and forever and that I would be able to cease having the Eligard.

It didn't work out that way. Eradicating cancer isn't readily achieved. It seemed that the cryotherapy didn't have much effect and in 2011 my PSA readings took off again, from 0.25 at the beginning of the year to 5.3 in the space of only 12 months.

Hormone Therapy

So it was back to hormone therapy again, this time for keeps: four-monthly Eligard injections, as before.

I was still very distressed at having to undergo this process and looking at the bruised area on my belly where the needle had gone in only made the feeling worse. It took quite a time for the understanding to sink in that there was absolutely no alternative; I simply *had* to accept my situation and make the best of it.

There was one ray of hope: I had read about *intermittent* hormone therapy and asked my urologist about this. He was happy for me to try it. It means suppressing the cancer by starving it of testosterone for a time, then ceasing the hormone injections altogether until the PSA level starts to climb again, indicating that the cancer is growing back once more. The idea is that with constant hormone dosage, the cancer will eventually become immune to it and begin its fatal spread through the body, whereas stop-start hormone treatment doesn't give the cancer sufficient time to develop this immunity. That's the theory as I understand it, anyway.

I believe strongly (largely because I *want* to believe this) that intermittent hormone therapy will keep me going longer than the continuous version. However, my urologist says that intermittent HT is not necessarily better, pointing out that (in his view) the pros and cons more or less cancel each other out, with continuous treatment doing a better job of suppressing the cancer but posing higher side-effect risks from heart trouble, depression and all the other things, while intermittent treatment isn't so good at suppression but lessens the side-effect dangers. This makes me feel that having future PSA monitoring tests at four-monthly intervals rather than the six months he suggested at first might be a better way of monitoring my situation and deciding in a more timely fashion when I might change from one regime to the other.

I have read other opinions that strongly back up the idea that intermittent hormone therapy appears to delay the change of the prostate cancer to a type that resists hormone therapy. If it does, the prostate cancer will be controllable for a longer period of time, as well as improve the quality of life. This is the view of Dr 'Snuffy' Myers, whose free internet talks and advice on all aspects of prostate cancer are a great source of information. He says, citing his long clinical experience, that intermittent hormone therapy, combined with a healthy lifestyle (right diet, plenty of exercise) can extend a man's life for a remarkably long time.

After resuming hormone therapy my PSA fell to below 0.4 and stayed around that level during the rest of 2012 and into mid-2013. On the basis of this, the urologist thought I could go off the hormone therapy at that point. So at the time of writing this account (September 2013) all I am doing is monitoring my PSA and hoping it will remain low for a year or more while I enjoy a spell from the side effects of the hormone therapy. Sooner or later, of course, the PSA will creep up again and hormone treatment will have to begin again.

Living with the Side Effects

Hormone therapy is certainly life-prolonging, but it comes with some major and unpleasant side effects. There is a tendency in some of the literature to underplay them or brush them aside, as though they don't matter all that much. We've all read notes about hospital procedures or medical treatments that say platitudinous things like, *Some patients may experience minor discomfort ...* The fact is, that while some side effects might be rather rare and/or not particularly severe, others are extremely serious and would be more accurately described as 'inevitable consequences' or 'inescapable collateral damage'.

I have experienced or am experiencing almost all the 'side effects' of hormone therapy that can be expected. It is difficult, though, to be certain whether what I think are side effects of the hormone therapy are entirely that or whether they are simply the result of getting old. Most likely both factors are at work.

Chemical Castration

No man likes the idea of being castrated, whether by chemicals, the surgeon's scalpel, flying shrapnel, barracuda attack, unfortunate meteorite impact or any other way. To me, castration was the most frightening 'side effect' of hormone therapy (although some of the others were pretty worrying as well) but by this time I'd accepted the fact of no other option – without hormone therapy the cancer would spread and I would die. So to stay alive I would have to undergo hormone therapy and the slow castration that went with it.

I don't recall any of the doctors I saw at the time taking much trouble to explain and discuss the matter in a sympathetic effort to soften the blow. I then spent a lot of time reading about it in the various handout booklets and pamphlets with a stomach-turning feeling about what was going to happen to me.

Body Changes

Once hormone therapy began, my genitals began to shrink away alarmingly; the hair disappeared from my chest and armpits and thinned out along my arms and legs. Nothing could be done about any of this. There was a moderate development of breast fattening – I thought it looked like the pectoral fat that middle-aged, elderly and overweight men easily get and I convinced myself that it wasn't very noticeable, at least if I was wearing clothes. I began to get a little tubbier than I had been before, although I wasn't really sure if this wasn't from eating too much. There was also a considerable loss of muscle mass – it took me a long time to realise that this was happening.

I didn't develop a high voice or turn into a woman, though. Nor did I even begin to feel like one. In fact I still feel very much like a man. I still look with interest at women on the trams, on the streets or on TV. Although my libido has plummeted and I am totally impotent, overall the chemical castration didn't bring on all the sickening and depressing outward physical and inner mental changes I'd been dreading.

One thing I found, after ceasing the brief spell on hormone therapy I had in 2009, was that stopping it didn't automatically reverse the bodily changes. There was a modest or partial 'un-castration' during the year I was off it, but it looked to me as though a lot of the hormone damage was going to be permanent. Perhaps there might have been a more complete recovery if I'd stayed off the hormones for longer but, back then, when my PSA shot up from 0.25 to 5.3 in a year, I didn't want to put off having hormone therapy any longer.

Impotence

Having sex is a very normal part of life but for me it is now ruled out altogether. I can make myself quite miserable if I'm silly enough to dwell on this, but I comfort myself by remembering that a lot of ageing couples just let sex fade out of their lives for all sorts of reasons. While I don't like this incapacity, I seem to have accepted it, by and large. My wife and I get by with cuddles, affectionate words and just being companionable, and lots of other couples do the same.

Osteoporosis and Heart Trouble

Among the other side effects are increased risks of osteoporosis, heart trouble and stroke. My urologist referred me to a specialist men's health team of endocrinologists and cardiologists at Austin Hospital. The object of this was to monitor and advise me as to how I was going with regard to these perils, and take whatever action was needed. A scan established that my bone density was at the lower end of the acceptable range and I'm countering this by taking the recommended Vitamin D3 tablets and Caltrate.

I also belong to a support group called Prostate Melbourne, which meets once a month at Royal Melbourne Hospital. Many of the men who come along are in much worse circumstances than me, and these meetings have given me a good perspective of my own state of affairs. Listening to other men there, in particular the chairman of the group, Wolfgang Schoch, convinced me to take up going to the gym regularly to give my bones a bit of work to do, to stop them getting any weaker and stop my muscles from fading away any further, while at the same time being good for the heart and general well-being.

Hot Flushes, Incontinence and Sleeplessness

Some of the men in my support group suffer very badly from hot flushes, but in my case I am fortunate that these flushes are not particularly troubling. I usually experience several hot flushes during the day, but they don't cause me to break out in copious sweats and I think a lot of minor ones pass unnoticed.

It's different at night, when hot flushes frequently wake me up. If I throw off the quilt to cool down, it's not long before I'm freezing and have to cover up again. Often these hot-flush wake-up calls coincide with the need to urinate – usually three times a night but sometimes more. Apart from that, I'm fortunate not to have any serious incontinence issues. I hope it stays that way.

Getting a good night's sleep is rare. Apart from the hot flushes and the need to go to the loo, I'm often disturbed by the rhythmic impacts of my artificial heart valve thudding away inside my chest. As well, my wife sleeping beside me often needs assistance with her breathing machine, which means taking sleeping pills is not on. So on the whole my sleep pattern is not good, and if I only have to get up three or four times a night, I regard that as a reasonable night's sleep.

Fatigue and Dizziness

I'm at my best in the mornings. By the afternoon I often feel weary and have a lie-down for half an hour or so. I have noticed that since I started going to the gym about six months ago, I have fewer afternoon lie-downs (although I still enjoy them when I do).

One thing that concerns me is that I often feel a little woolly-headed or giddy, and my sense of balance is faulty. This comes and goes, and when it's feeling bad I like to lean or hold on to something in case I fall over. I don't use a walking stick yet but I keep one ready by the door and another one in the car.

Brain Function

Over the last couple of years I have noticed my powers of concentration waning a little, and my short-term memory becoming unreliable. I have no idea whether this is a result of the hormone therapy or early stage Alzheimer's, or just simply old age. Quite possibly it's an amalgam of all three. I am finding this memory loss increasingly worrying but I don't think there's anything much I can do about it.

Valerie says that since going off hormone injections eight months ago, I am less vague and muddle-headed the way I often was while on the treatment. Going to the gym might be contributing to this improvement.

Putting on Weight

One of the well-known side effects of hormone therapy is a tendency to put on weight. This happens despite the accompanying loss of muscle mass and decreased bone density, so the gain must be all from extra fat. I firmly believe that eating (and drinking!) the right things in the right quantities, together with plenty of exercise and activity, will make this less of a problem. Unfortunately I like my own cooking, and so does Valerie, and that's one reason I have found it very hard to keep up the necessary resolve. It's all too easy to lapse back into old habits and let the weight pile back on again.

Depression

Contemplating death from prostate cancer must be as good a reason as any for feeling depressed. I sometimes feel I'm on the verge, but so far it hasn't become entrenched clinical depression and I can think of several reasons for this.

First and foremost is that Valerie and I have a very loving and very supportive relationship. She deserves heaps of credit for the fact that I don't get depressed. We have been married for 45 years. We like being together, we talk things over, make plans and decisions together, and we don't quarrel or bicker. If I need some gentle suggestions about getting through the daily jobs, she does it in the nicest possible way.

We have a few other good things going for us as well. We own our own apartment and our money worries are not huge. We have both led interesting lives and retained plenty of old friends from the different places and episodes in our past, and, to our great pleasure, our friends often come and stay with us. Our two sons – who live in remote corners of Australia – come to visit us occasionally. Our daughter and her family live just one suburb away and we see them often, including twice a week when I collect the two granddaughters from school and bring them home. They like us and we like them. Amusing and clever grandchildren are excellent antidepressants!

I have come to believe firmly that walking, exercising, going to the gym and just generally being active will keep me feeling good. Conversely, if I let the activity lapse and overeat and overdrink as well, I find myself becoming introverted and prone to gloomy thoughts. The psychological benefits of exercise and keeping active are well-documented, and I can verify this from my own experience.

Doing something creative puts me in a good mood. For the last eight years or so I have been writing short stories or little memoirs about things that happened to me over the years, so as to leave some knowledge about me to my descendants (assuming they bother to read them). I write about three or four of these a year. And I also do occasional (and very amateurish) acrylic paintings, usually of geological subjects, maybe one a year. Not a high production rate but I spend much more time thinking up the words and the designs than I do on the actual writing or painting, and that is part of the enjoyment and the benefit.

Talking with the Specialist

When I was first told I had cancer, apart from feeling shocked and frightened, I also felt powerless and utterly in the hands of the various specialists, busy men who tended to conduct rather short consultations, leaving me wishing there'd been more time for leisurely explanations and the opportunity to mull it all over and absorb all the unpalatable facts. These days, whenever I have an appointment with my urologist, I usually hand him a list of three or four written questions that I've thought of over the preceding weeks. If I don't put them down on paper, I'm bound to forget them and then be annoyed with myself when I remember them later. The first time I did this he was a little surprised, but now he *expects* me to provide a list of questions. We have a routine – while he is telling me the answers he also jots them down on the page, then he scans it into his files and gives it back to me for my own records. Not all doctors would welcome such questioning or respond so willingly, but my urologist does.

Sometimes I ask the same question on consecutive appointments. A favourite one is, 'Why are we assuming that my cancer is still encapsulated and not quietly spreading through my bones?' He makes his explanation and off I go home, feeling a little less worried.

Looking Ahead

Valerie came along in her wheelchair to meet my urologist one day. She remembers me asking him the question, 'How long will I live if nothing is done?' and his reply, 'About four years.'

That was well over four years ago. Despite all our physical troubles and constraints, Valerie and I go on living pretty good lives, all things considered. We know this can't go on indefinitely. Any day or night one of us could have a catastrophe – or even just some minor mishap – that will signal the end of our happy togetherness. In the meantime we are doing our best to stretch out this precarious but very agreeable existence. With any luck it'll be for a long, long time.

I'll Never Forget Jess Judge

Peter Laud

I'll never forget Jess Judge. Jess was the urologist who diagnosed my cancer and was the surgeon who, two months later, removed it. We met barely half a dozen times but I'll never forget the man with the soft, gentle handshake, the impeccable dark suit, and the slow and measured speech.

It came as a shock when Jess told me I had prostate cancer and that something needed to be done. Me, cancer? Surely not. Some error in the paperwork maybe? After all, my PSA was only 4.5 – not unusual for a bloke in his late 50s – and the specialist who did the biopsies had taken a preliminary look and indicated that there probably wasn't much to worry about. 'Go home and enjoy the holiday,' he'd said. It was Christmas Eve 1997.

Two weeks later on one of those boiling hot summer days that Perth specialises in, Jess sat in his air-conditioned room and said there was no mistake. The biopsies and the DRE had revealed what he called 'some activity' in the prostate gland.

I'd known something wasn't right. You don't go to the toilet six or seven times a night and pretend that everything is normal. After his diagnosis, I sought information from another specialist. The outlook was not good; my Gleason score indicated a rapid deterioration in quality of life within five years. I rang Jess the next day and he said that radical surgery seemed the best option and then endured six weeks of, *Why me?*

In the middle of the night, unable to sleep, I went for long moonlit walks in the hills east of Perth where we were living at the time. I overdosed on information about prostate cancer and how others had fared. I visualised my cancer as a black spider crouching somewhere within. Normally I quite like spiders but this one I wanted out and quickly.

After surgery I had an overwhelming feeling of relief. When the catheter was removed I asked to take it home minus the contents. I filled it with water, hung it up on a nail and gave my wife and each of our five kids a dart. The one who burst the catheter was rewarded with a Mars bar.

Three months of incontinence wasn't much fun. Pads helped but there's nothing like a pair of damp trousers to lower the spirit. I could have written a decent guidebook to just about every public toilet in Perth. And, as for erectile dysfunction, well, you can't have sex in a coffin.

I still go for my PSA test every six months and feel a rising tide of tension before each one. The results have been uniformly low. So, life goes on much as before, but a cancer diagnosis does change your outlook. I've been lucky. Lucky to have had the support of a loving family. Lucky to have been diagnosed in the first place when two GPs had said there was nothing to worry about. And lucky to have met the man in the dark blue suit with the fingers of a pianist. I'll never forget Jess Judge.

Rounding Up the Prostates

Judith O'Malley-Ford

He'll be rounding up the prostates when he comes,
He'll be rounding up the prostates when he comes,
He's a surgeon of urology, abnormal histology,
He'll be rounding up the prostates when he comes.

Oh, the prostate is a tricky little gland,
Oh, the prostate is a tricky little gland,
Oh, the prostate gland is tricky, it's a tricky little dickey,
Oh, the prostate is a tricky little gland.

Oh, the prostate never sees the light of day,
Oh, the prostate never sees the light of day,
Oh, the prostate is reclusive, and very much elusive,
Oh, the prostate never sees the light of day.

Oh, the prostate is the ruler of the man,
Oh, the prostate is the ruler of the man,
With lycopene protection, supplemented with affection,
Oh, the prostate is the ruler of the man.

Oh, the prostate gland it leads a life of shame,
Oh, the prostate gland it leads a life of shame,
Oh, the prostate gland will shame you; it will torture you
and maim you,
Oh, the prostate gland it leads a life of shame.

Oh, the moral to the story's very clear,
Oh, the moral to the story's very clear,
Prostates need attention, care, and intervention,
To avoid the consequences and the fear.

Connecting with the Specialists, Myself and My Feelings

Alan Raby

Aged 60, there was an abnormality in the paraprotein of my blood, an early indication something wasn't quite right. It took further analysis for the diagnosis to come back: Chronic Lymphocytic Leukaemia (CLL).

My GP recommended regular blood tests. Quarterly blood tests thereafter led to the discovery of a slightly elevated PSA a year later. As it turned out, the prostate would be the first cancer to be treated.

'It's probably the least bad cancer to have and usually something that people die *with* rather than *from*,' said one medically trained friend.

A friend called it a 'double whammy'. Detected early, I had two types of cancer and the treatment for the leukaemia would reduce my immune system and possibly allow the prostate cancer to grow.

I often ask myself what might have happened had it not been for my partner Lois. Had I been on my own, or had she been less knowledgeable, things might well have turned out differently for me.

It was she who insisted that, at 60, I have a thorough health check-up with my GP. This female GP was at first unwilling to give me a digital examination. I had just moved suburbs and was a new patient, but I insisted.

It's the first example of how we have had to challenge and insist since we knew from our research and advice that this was part of the methodology. It is all too easy to place our medical practitioners on a pedestal and take all their advice as gospel.

That is how my father was. He talked about his urologist in the NHS in the UK with personal sadness and regret. On his tour of the ward the day after surgery, the surgeon said to Dad, 'You were a tough old boot.' He was referring not to my father's physique, but the difficulty of the surgery. Dad had the distinct impression that the 'knife had slipped', leaving him incontinent. So for the rest of his 15 remaining years it was a life of social embarrassment, incontinence pads and mother telling him when he should change them. His sense of smell was already poor, so after she died he became more and more housebound, afraid of what others might think of his smell.

A year after my initial 'male health check-up' we moved from Sydney to Hobart. I had a referral from Sydney's St Vincent Hospital to the Royal Hobart Hospital for any follow-up treatment for the CLL. The only other thing we needed was a GP who was on our wavelength.

By asking friends and acquaintances we found Dr Sally Chapman MBBS FRACGP, who combined the western practice of medicine with these less mainstream lines of treatment. She is a member of the Australasian College of Nutritional and Environmental Medicine (ACNEM). Over the years we have established an informed dialogue with her. As a result, never expect Sally to be on time for her appointments. She takes as long as necessary in each consultation.

She arranged my follow-up blood tests for the CLL when I was 62. That was when my elevated PSA was first noticed. Her initial view was that an immediate radical prostatectomy might be the best approach for me. She recommended Michael Vaughan, a local urologist, (and member of the Urological Society of Australia and New Zealand).

Michael is one of a kind. For the next four years we would spend at least 20 minutes with him every 12 weeks and got to know him well. On the walls of his waiting room are paintings about a metre high done by his sons when they were in primary school, full of bright primary colours, with a Sydney Nolan look and feel. Quite impressive. I talked about my volunteer work on rites of passage for teenage boys and their families and he shared stories about his boys – now teenagers – and their achievements, like any other proud father.

At each consultation, Lois and I also improved our understanding and knowledge of prostate cancer. Michael explained the treatment options, which – for me – he considered to be a radical prostatectomy. Other options included brachytherapy (*but*, beware, he said, if the cancer is not cured this way, surgery afterwards is not an option. The tissues are too difficult to operate on after this local radiation). There was also the notion of 'active surveillance'. Because we were in a new relationship the sexual side of things was very important and the phrase 'nerve sparing' and its benefits were immediately of interest.

In one of our quarterly meetings, Michael once described nerve sparing from a surgeon's point of view like trying to carefully peel back a soggy facial tissue with surgeon's tools, remove the prostate, and then put all the tissue back without damaging any of the nerves. We got the point, and it was another step in our move towards a nerve-sparing robotic-assisted surgery.

I talked about my situation at a men's group I had just joined – one of the men who'd had a prostatectomy suggested I go to a meeting of the Prostate Cancer Support Group in Hobart.

Here I heard sagas from the men who, like my father, clearly had some issues after their surgery, some of it a decade earlier. These regular meetings were great for newcomers like me. It made me more determined to avoid their fate. I certainly paid careful attention to the visits of specialists about modern treatments.

One of them was local physiotherapist Jane Barker who spoke about the critical importance of pelvic floor exercises. This was one that Lois wanted to attend. (That's something else I noticed – in a group of a dozen men, there were never more than one or two wives/partners present. I never did find out how many of the men had partners or were living on their own.)

So after Jane's excellent talk with an illustrated PowerPoint presentation, we arranged a private session so that Lois could discover if I was contracting the right muscles. Using the same ultrasound machine that my urologist uses at my quarterly check-ups, she was able to confirm I was contracting my pelvic floor muscles. I have since watched a Prostate Cancer Support Group video that shows another method in which you see the flaccid penis move up slightly as the pelvic floor muscles are contracted.

Much relieved that I was doing it correctly, Lois was then forever reminding me to do my daily routine. Jane had recommended a set of ten slow contractions holding each one for ten seconds, a rest, ten quick contractions, a rest, and then repeat the ten ten-second contractions. It may have sounded like nagging in other situations, but those gentle reminders meant that I was soon doing it standing or sitting, as we were driving in the car, or in bed at night. My motivation came from meeting the challenge and the knowledge that I would be in fine shape for the surgery.

In November 2008, Michael performed a biopsy in which 14 cores were taken from my prostate via the perineum under a general anaesthetic. This was followed by a CAT scan to be certain that nothing had spread to the surrounding bones. The scan came back clear and we settled on 'active surveillance' since the PSA was showing no signs of doubling in 12 months.

Diagnosis: Stage T1C – T2A

Gleason score: 3+3 adenocarcinoma prostate

Treatment regime: Active surveillance November 2008 to July 2012 with quarterly PSA blood tests, digital rectal examination and ultrasound of prostate by urologist.

Lois and I would research online but most importantly in books. After reading and both of us marking up our copy of *Localised Prostate Cancer: A Guide for Men and their Families* (available from the Cancer Council in your state) I made some notes for our next consultation with Michael:

- Erectile dysfunction in general population is high anyway. So how does it compare with prostate sample?
- How many procedures have you done?
- What is my prognosis with my symptoms?
- What determines the wide range of erectile dysfunction after surgery? (30–90% is a huge range)
- Is robot-assisted surgery available in Hobart? Does it improve outcomes?
- Nerve sparing: how often have you done it? And what percentage of erectile dysfunction in your patients?
- Brachytherapy: this is erectile dysfunction of 50–55%. Correct?
  - How high is cost?
- Hobart versus Sydney versus Melbourne for treatment?

Then another quote in our reading hit us between the eyes:

> One US study showed the best results were achieved by surgeons who did more than 40 operations per year and hospitals which did more than 60 operations a year.

Looking back in my files I find one paragraph we marked. It kind of sums up my position:

> Men are less likely to have problems with erections after surgery if they have good sexual relations before the operation, are younger, their cancer is still small and a nerve-sparing operation has been used. A nerve-sparing operation is only possible if the cancer has not spread along the nerves.

We both wanted this kind of outcome. We asked Michael about robotic nerve-sparing options and he told us about John Yaxley in Brisbane, who performed hundreds of these procedures (many more than him) in a year, and how he had operated with John and could recommend the man. We asked for a referral and had an appointment with John in July 2011.

In response to our question about success rates John shared these post-operative figures:

- One third will get erections without assistance
- One third with assistance (e.g. Viagra)
- One third probably won't get erections after surgery.

We liked what we saw and heard and it was left up to me to decide when to have the robotic surgery.

Early in our relationship in 2002, Lois suggested I stop eating a lot of pre-packaged supermarket meals. My particular favourite was a delicious cheesy lasagne. When I cut back on this and many other very processed foods, it felt as if a 'fog' had lifted from my brain. It was the first of many experiences in which her advice had been useful.

So in 2008, I was very open to her ideas about how to proceed during this 'active surveillance'. Good nutritional food and a plethora of dietary supplements were our next line of defence against the slow-growing tumour. Lois bought me an Ian Gawler CD *Eating for Recovery*. In Sydney, we had been regular readers of free newspapers such as *Nova* (http://www.novamagazine.com.au/) and *Living Now* (http://www.livingnow.com.au/) and I already had a growing folder of articles on, say, the role of Vitamin D in maintaining the body's immune system. It was this system that we now set about improving as best we could. Lois put before me the benefits of a total detoxification of the body on a health farm and the notion of antioxidants. I declined the most radical ideas of a health farm, fasting or a detox regime on a health farm and focused on some of her other recommendations. Whatever the final treatment, if my body was at its optimum fitness, then I would recover more quickly with fewer side effects.

I started taking Vitamin C, our GP tested my Vitamin D (which was very low), and we added that to our daily supplements, along with lots of vegetables and fruit. A Mediterranean-style diet is perhaps the closest way to describe it. Salt and sugar – which many researchers say is part of the Western diet's problem and cancer causation – is hardly ever used. We don't use a supermarket or much processed food. Living in Tasmania, we do have a distinct advantage over the majority of urban dwellers. Home-grown veggies from the garden took on a new importance.

I spent a little more time in meditation using pre-recorded meditation CDs but it is not something that I find easy to make a regular part of my life.

I reduced my volunteer work and replaced it with gardening, bushwalking and other more physical activities. I stopped reading the newspapers or following the news of the day. Instead, I concentrated on the bigger picture and my mental state.

Most importantly, our love-making became more critical.

How did I feel during these years of 'active surveillance'? It's a question that Lois often asked me. I think I can recognise both optimism, and then disappointment that my dietary changes and supplements did not make the cancer shrink and disappear. My reading had included books by Louise Hay and the like who claim that 'alternative' methods have 'cured' their cancers.

Part of me liked the idea of the body being able to heal itself if the conditions are right, but as I thought about it, even Ian Gawler had initially used Western treatments and turned to 'alternative' things afterwards to keep himself healthy. Maybe that would be my approach.

Each quarter, with only slight variations up or down, my PSA reading was pretty stable. It was not doubling in 12 months, which – according to Michael – would have been cause for concern. My readings fluctuated over the course of the next year, although there was a steady increase. Then, by late 2011, my GP noticed that my CLL was becoming an issue. I had no symptoms at that time, but my haemoglobin (red blood cell count) and my platelets were going down. I was referred to Dr Rosemary Harrup, an oncologist in Hobart, and she made it clear that the chemotherapy regime for me (three drugs given monthly as an outpatient over three days known as FCR) had a fair chance of success. It was well-researched and gave good remission rates. However, these drugs were immunosuppressive and the prostate could then become more aggressive and a danger. It had to be treated first.

I delayed and delayed since, at that time, I felt no CLL symptoms. Then, slowly, I realised that I was getting breathless doing gardening. I had already *not* taken Michael Vaughan's advice to have a second biopsy in 2010, which is part of 'active surveillance'. I'd had slight post-operative pain in the perineum after the biopsy in 2008, it would cost another $1,000, and I rationalised that the PSA readings were enough of a measure.

Finally, when Lois was away on a meditation retreat I read from cover to cover *Prostate Cancer: Your Guide to the Disease, Treatment Options & Outcomes* (3rd Edition 2010 by Prem Rashid). It lays out the science and treatment options like a school textbook with summaries at the beginning and end of each chapter. I thoroughly recommend it. My passage of urine was getting much slower, although with no pain; I felt it was time to book that surgery in Brisbane.

We would need to be there a week beforehand to allow John Yaxley to organise an MRI to give him an up-to-date view of the prostate, plus some tests on my breathing (the CLL condition) and to have a backup oncologist see me. Since we needed to allow for a post-operative week while the catheter was in, we arranged it as one week for the treatment 'bookended' with one week of holiday either side as tourists in Brisbane. I thoroughly recommend the approach to reduce the stress and to create a healing environment.

Surgical removal of prostate July 2012

Robotic-assisted laparoscopic radical prostate

PSA after operation < 0.05

It was a long six-and-a-half hour procedure and I had six units of blood due, most likely, to the CLL condition. Yet, there was a salutary lesson for me as I remember some details in John Yaxley's post-operative consultation before we flew back to Hobart.

This machine is accurate to 0.05mm, he said, and he had to do some very fine work around the back of the prostate where the cancer had almost broken out. So, by not having the biopsy in 2010, and trusting in the PSA alone, there but for the grace of God I had almost left the decision to operate too late. If John had not reported back that the 'margins were clear' I might have had to have radiation to kill lingering cancer cells.

As I write this (October 2013) my PSA is still <0.05 and I have just successfully completed a six-month course of FCR chemotherapy for the CLL.

I look ahead to many more years of contented, active retirement.

My Special Saint

Richard Stone

'Better get "it" in while you can, Kenny.' He followed that with a conciliatory, 'You'll be right.'

How would he bloody well know I would be 'right'? Right about what? Why do people say that when they must know the situation is far from being 'right'? Another bright spark, complete with a repeating bending finger gesture, laughingly whispered, 'Drip, drip, drip.' I'm glad he was amused. Further advice was, 'Shouldn't that type of news be kept in the family?'

Great mates! Why did I bother telling them anything after my visit to the urologist? My appointment had been a few days earlier when the specialist had informed me, 'I'm sorry, Mr Williams, Ken, but your biopsy proves my suspicions. You have prostate cancer. Your Gleason Score is six which means we must take a course of action.'

My wife Jenny told me later that my face was ashen. I don't know about that. I do recall the ringing in my ears and the deeply sinking feeling in my gut. I wanted to vomit. Held it back by breathing rapidly.

Jenny took over (thank heavens my saint was there; I was speechless for a time). 'What's the next move, doctor?' she asked.

'Well, obviously Ken will need to have the cancer treated. There are a number of options for treatment. At the end of this visit, I'll provide you with information concerning the various treatments available.'

'Could you give us an overview of the various treatments now please, Doc?' I managed to squeeze out.

'Well now, there is of course a radical prostatectomy which is the removal of the prostate gland and a few lymph nodes from around that area. We consider that to be the "gold standard" treatment. There are low dose and high dose radiation treatments. A relatively new and largely experimental treatment, High Intensity Focussed Ultra Sound, is available but only in major city centres. However, HIFU is also rather expensive and not fully covered by Medicare or private health funds. Then there is hormone treatment. Lastly, there is the method of "watchful waiting". This is a controversial treatment for younger men because waiting too long could allow the cancer to escape the prostate gland.'

'Wow, Doc, which treatment do you advise? I had no idea there were so many options.'

'As you are in your early 60s and fit with no other diseases evident, you are considered to be young in terms of prostate cancer treatments. I suggest you study these brochures and return within a week to discuss further your preferred treatment option. You might also glean information from the internet from accredited medical sites.'

'Does the biopsy reveal the extent of the cancer? Can it tell if the cancer has escaped from the prostate gland?'

'We won't know the extent of the problem until the prostate is removed and examined by a pathologist. In any event, there are follow-on treatments for cancer beyond the gland. Let's discuss the matter at your next appointment, after you've had time to examine the information. Feel free to seek a second opinion. In the meantime, I'll arrange for a few necessary blood tests and bone and CT pelvic scans for you.'

I now had a week to reflect on my predicament – the *Big* C. Now it was personal, now it was *me*. I remembered nodding sympathetically when I'd heard of others with cancer, both male and female. But let me be honest, I'd made an inward sigh of relief that it wasn't me and carried on with whatever I was about. I was bloody fearful now – no use denying it. A fair bit of self-pity reigned, the old *why me?* syndrome. I also experienced a truckload of anxiety. Jenny was attuned to my fear and trepidation.

'Look, Kenny, we've been through heaps together. We won't let this beat us, Darls. I'll tell the kids you need a "waterworks" operation. No sense in worrying them too much. Let's study the info and see if we can make a treatment decision.'

Still, I was filled with trepidation and wanted the week to pass quickly towards my next specialist visit. I had trouble sleeping. I also found difficulty in erasing the thought of a possible raging cancer invading my body from that troublesome walnut-sized gland. Nevertheless, I had to make a decision. Jenny and I talked the matter through.

'I've decided to go with the radical prostatectomy, Doc.'

'Fine. I'll schedule an operation for the week after next. My receptionist will give all the information before you leave today. Let me ask you a question. What is your biggest fear regarding the procedure?'

'I'm mostly fearful of being incontinent and I'm not too happy about being impotent either.'

'All urologists are adept at nerve-sparing techniques that can affect the functions you mention. That said, however, there is a chance of incontinence and also a high degree of probability that there will be some form of erectile dysfunction, an inability to have or maintain an erection naturally. Sometimes the ED aspect is dependent on the quality of erections before the operation.'

'I've read that there are methods to overcome these problems.'

'Indeed there are. You will be incontinent for about six weeks after the operation. You will need to wear pads for this time. Have you been performing the pelvic floor exercises?'

'Religiously. Every day.'

'Good. We can assess the situation after six weeks. I assure you that there have been marvellous developments in effectively fixing incontinence problems. Concerning ED, there are a number of techniques. Viagra and Cialis can be tried to improve an erection. Should those medications fail, one can inject a solution into the penis shortly before intercourse.'

'Ouch! That sounds painful.'

'Surprisingly it's not a painful method. Also, a vacuum pump can be used to induce an erection. The erection is maintained by the use of a rubber ring. Finally, a prosthesis can be inserted into the cavities of the penis. The device is surgically implanted and is operated by fluid from a small internal pump. The pump is operated by squeezing on a specific part of the device.'

Decisions on which procedure to adopt could wait. I needed to get through the next phase first, the radical prostatectomy.

A week later, and after scans revealed the cancer was not evident elsewhere, I sat on the end of the bed nervously awaiting the trolley trip to the operating theatre.

My wife, waiting with me, soothed, 'You'll be right, Darls.'

There was that inane statement again but at least I got a cuddle and a kiss with it from my saint.

Celebrating MOvember

Judith O'Malley-Ford

On the first of MOvember
as you will remember
it's time for each man to stand tall

till December at last, with gigantic moustache
from his lip to the end of the mall

Don't Pass 'GO'

Morgan Flint

I moved to Adelaide at the beginning of 2008, and almost immediately started to experience pain in the lower abdomen. I put the pain down to adjustment to a new, floor-level bed.

In April I went to see a GP. Dr PC (who runs two patients at a time!) couldn't see very much wrong. It wasn't until after a few more visits that he thought perhaps a bit of testing was called for.

To cut a long story short, scans suggested something more serious than simple abdominal/back pain. Tests over the next few months strongly suggested that my prostate was the cause of the problem.

He referred me to JM, a urologist, who arranged a biopsy on my prostate. The result was a Gleason score of eight and radical surgery was suggested, to which I agreed.

Earlier, I must have had a blood test, and the PSA level would/must have shown the presence of cancer, hence (I guess) the scans.

Dr PC, at no stage, suggested anything other than surgery, which after my experience, I now know to be quite unacceptable; I should have been given options to consider. Nor did he point out to me that there was no need to rush into a decision.

The operation was carried out on 24 March 2009. The following day, JM stated that he 'had got it all'.

Within a day or so, my urine was an odd colour. The nurses agreed.

JM was rather dismissive of my observation at first, but he soon came to see that a slip of the scalpel had caused a fistula.

Thus began a bloody awful year. I had about six operations and walked around with catheters, one in my penis and another draining my poo. I had an ileostomy, which, with the catheters, isolated the bowel and bladder so that the fistula could heal. I had to change the two bags every two or three days.

What really annoyed me was the change in my abdomen shape because this led to problems in the seal between my body and the bags. On more than one occasion, I woke to leaking fluids. There was a period when I had to change the bags four times in a day – really distressing.

In October 2009, I finally had the reversal done. Post-surgery at Calvary was both extremely painful and distressing. I had to have shots of morphine, so intense was the pain at times. I was also moved to a private room because I had pseudomonas, which is highly contagious.

About three weeks later, I had an intense pain in my lower abdomen. I couldn't move for about five minutes until it passed. Thinking it could be a post-ileostomy-reversal-operation-related condition, I rang Marian at the surgeon's rooms, and she said that if it were to happen again, I was to get an ambulance to hospital, ASAP.

The following morning I had to take her advice, and went to Ashford where I asked for a PSA reading to be done on the blood test which the doctor wanted done as part of his examination. This time, the pain was caused by a kidney stone.

That is when I learned two things about my health. Firstly, that I still had cancer, because my PSA was not zero and secondly that a PSA reading had been done while I was in hospital for one of my many earlier operations (June, in fact) and was found to be three. JM should have seen that, but if he had, he had done nothing!

I had one more consultation with JM, by which time the PSA had reached 12. His solution was to wait until it reached 30. (Was he effing serious?)

It was then that I decided to see an oncologist.

In early February, when my PSA had doubled from five to ten, this prompted Susan, my Alice Springs GP, to refer me to Ganeesan in Adelaide. I saw him on the 11th, at Daws Road, and he put me on to Casodex, because the Zoladex obviously wasn't doing its job. (Ganeesan is his shortened Indian name). He also ordered bone and CT scans and made an appointment for me to see a radiotherapist, just in case I would need it later.

I saw Tony Woo and he had the results of the PSA, and scans. There was a spot on my spine (T9–T10), which the scan report described as 'suspicious'. Tony also made the observation that there was cancer in my blood, and that this could have been there before the operation in March 2008.

He also said a Gleason score of eight meant that radiotherapy could have been an alternative to surgery. And not for the first time, I regretted not being referred to an oncologist instead of a urologist. That is the big lesson I learned out of this whole experience.

I then returned to G'nesh (an even shorter version of his name). The news was delivered in a much more sober manner.

In short, he did not pursue Tony's observation that there was cancer in my blood, but gave me medication to fix that. He noted the 'spot on the spine' comment from the radiotherapist, and said that at the first sign of back pain, I should contact them. Therefore, there was no reason why I shouldn't go to Europe for four months, as I had planned.

I now have prostate cancer, with secondaries in my ribs, spine and hip, and that has been situation for about four years.

Reflections/Conclusions

It was my uplifting meeting with Tony Woo that made me realise I should have gone directly to an oncologist as soon as cancer was diagnosed, *not* to a surgeon/urologist, because radiotherapy might have solved the problem and saved my vascular bundles.

I think all GPs need to give patients diagnosed with prostate cancer all the options for going forward, and not rush them into a decision.

I believe that each of us in a Prostate Support Group should document our personal experiences, and that they should go on file. Those experiences should let prospective cancer sufferers know what we have learned, and show any reservations or criticisms we have about our treatment.

We should also establish links with the GPs in Central Australia, with the view to having them refer all their patients diagnosed with cancer to our group; I know what I'll tell them – go straight to an oncologist. Don't pass GO. Go straight to the top.

Better still, get into the public health system, and be advised by a team of specialists – oncologist, dietician, radiotherapist, urologist, etc.

Clearing My Mind

Garry Wardle

There is no easy way to begin this journey.

There is ignorance within the general macho-male population about the reproductive system and its workings. All males need to know is that a yearly PSA blood test when over the age of 50 is *so* important. Early diagnosis of a prostate problem is imperative for a chance of defeating prostate cancer.

Diagnosis

It was early January 2008 during a doctor's visit for bad sinuses when I suggested a full check-up for someone my age (59). After donating a blood sample I forgot all about the tests, but some days later I received a phone call from the doctor saying he wanted to see me urgently.

This is not good, I thought.

This was the first of the many hurdles I would face, including the invasiveness of a rectal examination – a far from pleasant experience. Some of the best advice that came to mind was, *Keep biting your tongue and think of King and Country*. Afterwards, the doctor told me that my PSA was 4.2 and he could feel a lump in my prostate. I was to see a urologist urgently.

At the first appointment with the urologist, my wife Jenny and I were asked a myriad of sexual relationship questions. We were shown in detail what the problem was and given explanations to all the questions that came to mind. I was also given the names of other doctors to get second opinions. My head was spinning when I left the surgery and I am thankful that Jenny was with me to remember the details.

At the second opinion, I was asked to arrive with a full bladder, and to piddle into a funnel in the toilet. I wondered why but did as I was told. The first questions the doc asked were, do I have any problems with my water works and what about the urine flow? To which I answered that all is good and I have no real problems and that the last time I checked I could pee to head height. While referring to graph results from the funnel test he told me that this was not the case, and that I did have a flow problem. He explained the 'ins and outs' and said that reduced flow was not often noticed as the restriction of the urethra was very gradual, happening over a long period of time and more so as we get older.

Of course, the first thing I did when I got home was to fill up with water again and proceed outside to do my own test. I could not even get to nipple height much less over my head. This was a huge shock. If you manage to notice any change and believe things are not what they used to be, I cannot stress the importance of getting a check-up. However, keep in mind reduced flow does not necessarily mean there is a serious problem; there can be other reasons.

I made another appointment with the first urologist to finalise the next stage and to ask more questions. He booked me into hospital for a biopsy of the prostate, and explained that the procedure would involve taking samples from the prostate through the wall of the rectum. Upon seeing my face, the urologist explained that this procedure would be done while I was under sedation. He also told me that after the biopsy I could continue with normal sexual relationships within a few days, but not without a condom and that it would be better for me to masturbate for the next couple of weeks, as there would be some blood in my ejaculate until things healed. It was at this time that I made my first slight deviation from the truth with Jenny as to what the doctor really said.

Biopsy

The biopsy procedure was uneventful and I was back on the golf course in a few days. A couple of days later, I convinced Jenny that she had better see if everything was still working. Unfortunately this one-sided love affair concluded with the unforgettable expression of horror on her face when she saw the colour of my ejaculate. It took two weeks to settle down and a further week or so until I was allowed to go bareback again.

After the biopsy I visited my urologist for the verdict: 'I am sorry to tell you that there is cancer present. You have clinical cancer stage T2 with a Gleason score of seven'.

Jenny broke down and I was in shock. He booked me in for bone scan and CT scans to make sure the cancer had not spread. He told us I had some options as to my treatment, but his recommendation was to remove the prostate. He told me to study a booklet of information for a few weeks and get a second opinion from another surgeon specialising in radiation treatment if I wanted. When I had made my decision as to what course of action I wanted, I would go back and see him.

I do not want to understate the seriousness of later stage prostate cancers and the potential outcomes of men diagnosed with them. I soon learned that mine was at a stage that was treatable, with a good chance of cure, and my story continues with my heartfelt sympathies for those diagnosed with later stages of the disease.

For two weeks I read, but my mind was in turmoil. I read again, I surfed the net, but I was more confused than ever. Why did they give me the options? I was not qualified. But then I realised that I *was* qualified; it is my life, and, more importantly, my sexual life, a fact that I believe would be hard for any man to consider not having.

So I set myself a path of trying to understand the sexual workings of the male body and mind. Most men will have, at best, a very simplistic view of the relationships between orgasms, urinary tracts, nerves, penises, testes, ejaculations, erections and sperm. Like me, they will have had no idea that ejaculate is the mixture of sperm (none, if you have had a vasectomy, as I have had) from the testes and fluid from the prostate and seminal vesicles. Or that erections are a result of penile blood flow with intact penile nerves with or without stimulus triggered from the brain, or that orgasms are in the brain only, and have little to do with the penis.

It was with much trepidation that I came to understand most of the intricacies of this amazing machine all men worship but don't really understand. Yes, the doctors will go into all the diagrams, prognoses and technical jargon for you, as though it is just another broken down motor car, but let me tell you it isn't as simple as that when it is *your* body.

Decisions

It was then that I set myself up an excel spreadsheet to try and get all the critical information, side effects and percentages onto one sheet of paper so as to see and better understand the consequences of the next steps I would take on this journey. I basically had to make a decision between pretending that I was an ostrich and sticking my head in the sand, having a nerve-sparing radical prostatectomy (removal of the prostate but leaving some nerves behind if they can), or going with Brachytherapy (implants of radioactive seeds into the prostate). These three options were across the top of the page, and down the page were various consequences of these options: life span, various sexual effects (particularly that I would not have any more ejaculations), limited erections, probable urinary incontinence and rectal problems. This system, at least, got all the reams of paper I had read onto one page.

It was then that my worst fears of not being able to make Jenny's eyes pop again really struck home. This totally unfounded male assumption was a driving force behind my every thought, and, together with my selfishness of maybe losing my libido, it became all-consuming. I made no apologies for my relentless pursuit of wanting sex. Intimacy was seldom at the front of my mind; ejaculation was. Jenny was understanding; without her, life would have been far more troubled. Twenty-odd years of acting like rabbits might soon come to an end.

At this point in time I still did not comprehend that ejaculation and orgasm were separate, but related-functions, and that orgasm was not reliant on ejaculation. If I fully understood this moot point I may have had less apprehension and been able to have made decisions more quickly. I probably also would have understood women a bit more, as Jenny tells me time and time again – it's the brain you have to work on.

For some time I kept procrastinating and thinking that Brachytherapy was the way to go – the easiest way out of this jam. Then it was out on the golf course again within days. Jenny kept saying to go with the nerve-sparing radical prostatectomy. But, having lost a lot of money gambling in my earlier years and not having won a thing in my life worth talking about, I didn't like the odds. Small, I know, but when your life becomes odds you know in your heart you must back the favourite. In the end, I had to make a decision, and make an appointment with my GP, who I had known for some thirty years and who is now a surgeon. He had all the information at hand from both urologists, and, as I had the greatest respect for him, I told Jenny I would go with whatever he said.

His advice was direct: 'Get it out *now*. You have two school-age children and you and Jenny will adapt sexually if the worst happens.'

The next stage of the journey was all-consuming: decisions made, affairs in order, final dinners and romance out of the way; anyone would think I was going to the electric chair. The children asked questions, but, thankfully, the answer of having an operation to remove some cancer was all they needed.

The surgeon explained again exactly what he had planned. He would not promise any final outcomes, as it was dependent on what he would find when he opened me up and what was found when the prostate specimen had been analysed by the pathologist afterwards. My life was about to change big-time – hospital, here I come. Maybe a bit melodramatic, but with all the unknowns in this world of high-tech medical achievements I felt very vulnerable, but calm. It is amazing how, once I made my decision, the panic and anxiousness dissipated.

The Operation

I was in hospital the night before the early morning operation. As I was about to be wheeled to the theatre there was panic within the nursing ranks as I answered 'no' to the question, 'Have you been shaved?' This is where my inhibitions started to break down with nurses grabbing my essential bits and doing a record-breaking shave.

I woke up the next morning with a 100mm-long vertical scar under my navel, which was a surprise as I thought it would be horizontal. Next morning, the physiotherapist arrived and announced that we were off on our first walk.

Bloody hell, I thought. *Things are sore – you have to be joking. And what about this thing hanging out of my penis – a catheter. That's right, the surgeon mentioned this was going to be here for about ten days.*

I walked that first day unassisted, except for a walker, and further every day afterwards. Embarrassments faded very quickly and in no time I was doing laps around the nurse's quarters. Laughing was not an option; showering and the changing of bandages was not a pretty sight; but life got better rapidly.

The surgeon and the Sister-in-Charge checked me out the day after the operation and were very pleased with how the operation had gone. Some nerves were able to be saved as planned. The surgeon then proceeded to tell me, after the catheter was out, to feel free to give *him* a good slap around as often as possible to see how the erections would be. I don't know if I was embarrassed but I laughed out loud (ouch!) as I had never heard this euphemism before. However, the surgeon should have clarified his instructions as they had unexpected consequences.

The next stop was home. Jenny picked me up from hospital with all the attachments. The catheter was more annoying than anything else and sleeping was difficult. I learned a catheter is a tube that placed up through the urethra and into the bladder. A balloon is inflated inside the bladder to stop the catheter coming out. The urine continually runs into a bag (usually lying on the floor), that you empty every few hours. It is there to allow enough time for the anastomosis (join) between the bladder and urethra to heal.

On about the fourth morning of being home I had a frightful experience; it is not good to wake up with a quarter of an erection with a catheter in. Things very quickly dissipated and I began to understand that my future life may not be that bad after all.

Catheter

Ten days later we were back at the hospital to have the catheter taken out. The doctor explained that the urologist wanted the anastomosis tested with the catheter left in, but the balloon deflated. In the next breath he told me that voiding around the catheter would be highly unlikely to work, as he had only had a few successful tests in his career. He attempted to contact my surgeon to clarify his instructions but could not. Half an hour later, we decided to attempt the procedure, but by this time I was very apprehensive. First up, while I was lying down, he attached my catheter to a saline drip bag hanging about a metre above me, deflated the balloon inside my bladder, and slowly proceeded to fill my bladder. The doctor told me to yell when my bladder was really full, which was when he would turn off the tap, and get me on my side to piddle into a basin. Easy? Wrong; you have two nurses and a doctor watching and listening from nearby and you are lying down in a strange clinical environment. I was in pain for about 15 minutes when they came to check.

'No go,' I told them. 'Why haven't you got waterfall music playing?'

'Do you want to give it more time?' they asked.

'Yes.'

This time I relaxed and thought of that waterfall. A few minutes later there was a geyser as all was released. The doctor was impressed with my display, checked the x-rays and told me this wouldn't hurt a bit as he grabbed me 'old feller' and slowly pulled out the catheter.

As I walked out the door I thought, *God, it feels good to be free again.*

The next stage of this journey was that I relayed the doctor's 'slapping' instructions to Jenny, replacing the word 'me' with 'you' in the translation. It was with much trepidation that I ventured into this next stage. Yes, I could orgasm, but things were not the same, as I was filled with all the wrong thoughts. It was going to be a long road ahead.

It was also during this time that my apprehensions at the lack of having all the necessary 'hard drive' equipment started to eat away at my subconscious. Yes, I could get a partial erection, but it was not good enough to allow penetration.

From my point of view – maybe mistakenly – the ability of a man to have intercourse is a prerequisite to intimacy. Do not underestimate my anxiety at not being able to perform adequately. It was now that we needed to start exploring avenues that would allow me to do the deed.

Results

The doctor asked that I get a PSA test about six weeks after leaving the hospital. A few days after the test, Jenny and I went to see him. The results were not good. The Histology showed that the tumour was outside the prostate, abutting two margins (the area near the outer side of the prostate). There was also metastatic (spread) into the seminal vesicles. The PSA reading was low, but not low enough. After discussing whether I was incontinent and wearing pads, I answered in the negative but explained that I would occasionally have little accidents if I got tired. The next question he asked: 'Have you been getting erections?'

It was then I let him know what his instructions were and relayed how religiously we had been following those instructions. He then gave me another PSA form to check in one month's time, and told me not to have sex for the five days before the next PSA test.

The next couple of weeks were not a happy time, as I was expecting, and hoping that all would be clear. Later we went back in to see him but the results were still not what he would have liked. In fact, the PSA reading had increased. There were never any promises that surgery would cure my cancer, and the next stage of this journey began with an appointment to see a radiologist.

Radiation

Off I went to see a Radiation Oncologist. The doctor explained everything he was going to do together with the side effects. He booked me in to have my tattoos placed, one on each side of my hips and one about 75mm below my navel. These small tattoos would guide the position of the radiation beam with a very high accuracy to the area they want to treat, i.e. where the prostate was removed.

One week later I received the first of 35 radiation treatments. This procedure was painless and administered with a computerised machine that looks as if it belongs in *Star Trek*. I got six zaps of about ten seconds, each from various angles around my hips, and was then sent on my way. It was after about five weeks that the side effects start to hit. To be blunt, I did not know whether I wanted to crap, piddle or fart and, as a result, spent a large portion of my waking moments either sitting on the crapper or lying in a saltwater bath to lessen some of the consequences. Bladder control was also becoming painful. So, all in all, the radiation treatment did become debilitating towards the end and for two weeks after the last treatment, but not so much that it stopped me playing golf once a week. However, I now know every tree intimately on the golf course and the whereabouts of the two halfway toilets (exactly to the second at my sprinting pace). I did start taking a binding agent and an antacid drink, which helped alleviate the painful symptoms but not the number of visits.

Solving My Performance Problems

On a visit to the urologist, I explained the apprehensions I was having about sexual performance. The urologist prescribed Cialis and told me that it may improve the erections. This drug is very similar to Viagra, and over the next few weeks I tried this drug in various doses. The side effects were too much in that it swells my sinuses more than the intended object, and I felt so crook with headaches and hot flushes for 12 hours afterwards that it was not worth the trouble.

On a later visit to the urologist, he advised we should now consider other measures – maybe books, penile rings or injections. So off to a sex shop Jenny and I went; on the shopping list were books, rings for me, a vibrator, and a movie. Somehow, we would sort my problems out, but these remedies did not work, and, in my head, I believed there was still a lot missing. I was not a happy chappie, but Jenny was patient.

It was now that I knew I would have to get my head around the last throw of the dice – injections. I had read about these injections, and had discarded them due to being very afraid of needles, especially as it must be administered by Jenny or me and into a part of my anatomy that is very sacred.

After relaying some of the problems I was having to the Radiation Oncologist, he gave me the number of a Men's Clinic where all these problems could be solved. I rang and made an appointment. Jenny and I fronted up and went into the doctor's office where – and I will use Jenny's terms – she felt like she had 'the plague'. After a few minutes, Jenny got the hint and excused herself, and then it was down to secret men's business. The doctor was very professional and asked all the questions that no human had asked me before. After briefly explaining the procedures and warning me that I might experience extreme embarrassment, he asked if I wanted to proceed. I told him I doubted he could embarrass me after 59 years and the invasiveness of my experiences during the last eight months, so let's go.

Firstly, he explained everything in detail, including that the erection I would experience was entirely mechanical and I would have no control over it. This, I thought, I could handle fairly comfortably. He then did a detailed examination of my friend, which was very disconcerting for a minute. Then we went through the mechanics of using a syringe. This got my mind well and truly back on the task at hand, thankfully. He explained that you had a choice of either manual injections or using an applicator. There was no question which way I was going. We then proceeded to another room where everything was explained in detail again and I proceeded to inject a dose of liquid into the spongy tissue of my valued friend using the applicator. There was no pain; the smallest of pinpricks was all that was experienced, and I was then instructed to lie down for ten minutes or so. After this time, I was instructed to stand up; unbeknownst to me, things had definitely improved in sight only. The doctor and I were impressed, but he was not entirely happy and asked me to lie down again. He handed me a big dollop of lubricant and told me to see if I could do any better – but not to get *too* excited. He left the room and came back five odd minutes later to find things had vastly improved. He was now happier and I was also more than impressed. Doctor then explained that the erection would last for some time and if it didn't subside within 20 minutes to take one of two pills he gave me. If it still had not subsided after a further 20 minutes I would need to take the other one, and if it was still erect after another 15 minutes I would need to ring him. He then instructed me to wash up, get dressed and pick up my supply of syringes, needle disposal box, antiseptic pads, a vial of the magic potion and the applicator from the receptionist on the way out.

I now had a very challenging experience in front of me: how would I get out of here in this state? Luckily, I wore a loose-fitting shirt over a pair of jeans with a belt. I strapped him up and left the shirt out. I stood at the crowded reception area, awaiting my supplies. I also very quietly instructed Jenny to stand very close to me and to not move too far away.

My self-consciousness ran rampant as we made our way out the door and to the café next door, where I decided to sit and have a coffee and see what would happen. Nothing happened after 20 minutes, so I swallowed the first pill. I then believed things were going to literally greater heights and it was also becoming very painful. We decided to make our way down the street to the car, with me believing every person was looking at me as I strolled very closely behind Jenny. A twenty-minute drive later and five minutes from home, I was still in great discomfort, with my trousers and belt open. If the police had stopped me for any reason it would have been interesting to see how I would have gotten out of my predicament. I took the second pill and, 20 minutes later, I rang the doctor, but he was out and would ring me back.

I can tell you, the last thing I felt was sexy or aroused; in fact, quite the opposite was true. Ten minutes later, the doctor rang back, but things had started to subside and he instructed me to use smaller doses and to experiment with the doses until I felt comfortable with the results. This was one the most harrowing experiences of my life and, at this time, I was wondering if my two hundred-odd dollars had been wasted.

As it turned out, using injections was one of my best decisions. Yes, there were a lot of nervous trials and tribulations with getting the injection applicator to work and I guess if you had a third hand things may have been easier. Jenny refused to get involved with the mechanics, as it presented a foreplay-related emotional issue, I believe. After five goes I could inject comfortably and had the dose down to a third of what the doctor used on that fateful trial day.

Quickies on the kitchen bench were not an option and timing was everything for me. Twenty-odd minutes after injecting until action time, with a performance window of about twenty minutes. Jenny and I were back playing rabbits, but without the wet spots, and I could not be happier with the injections and would recommend them to anyone with a similar problem. Sometimes I experienced pain within the base of my penis after orgasm, but was told not to worry, as stretching scar tissue was the culprit. I still had misgivings about the orgasm side of things, but was assured over time, things should improve if old age didn't catch up to me first. I did miss my ejaculate, though.

Final Diagnosis

The last stage of my incredible journey was mid-October 2009; I had been given a very good report with my PSA down to .07 and stable. The doctor said that the reading should go lower over time and, other than six-monthly check-ups, my life can get back to normal.

In finishing, I may or may not have gotten rid of this life-threatening disease – there are no promises – but hopefully I will get a few more additional years out of this body.

Postscript

I would like to thank my wife Jenny; she has had her own problems with two separate mastectomies in the preceding seven years. Her unfailing love, support, encouragement and level-headedness have been an inspiration. My heart goes out to those who have far greater medical problems than I and I truly hope someone benefits from my diatribe – be it a laugh or the impetus to go and do something about any water-works problems without embarrassment. Please, men, I reiterate, go to your doctor and get your PSA check done today, as an early diagnosis is imperative.

Understanding

Ron Turner

Society dictates
I wear a mask,
hide my feelings strong,
play the part.

Myself,
not recognised
as I move from mood to mood,
to play the part.

I act in
so many roles,
no longer recognising me.
I play a part.

Remove the mask
so I might feel
that which is self.
What is my part?

Be quiet
and feel my peace,
giving love.

Be quiet
and feel my part;
     my part is love.

A Gay Man's Journey

Tony

My journey began in May 2010 when my regular six-monthly check-up showed a higher than usual PSA. (My GP said the rate of increase was more important than the actual level). He suggested seeing a urologist, who said I should have a biopsy but 'not to worry as prostate cancer is the most over-treated of cancers.' It was quite a shock, then, to get the results and find that nine of twelve samples showed cancer. The urologist said my Gleason score was 4+3. There was also a third 'score', which I've forgotten, but seemed to be serious. I staggered out of his surgery without paying the bill.

This diagnosis was a huge shock – bigger than a mild heart attack a year earlier. Up till then I had thought only other people got cancer. I lived a very healthy lifestyle in a very healthy environment and there was no cancer in my immediate family.

I sought two more opinions and finally punched the numbers into the excellent Memorial Sloan-Kettering Prostate Cancer website (www.nomograms.mskcc.org). This website talked about 'indolent' cancers, which would be 'watch and wait', although it said 'indolent' was not applicable in my case and gave the chances of dying from cancer within a various number of years. This agreed with my urologist who said that I was 'outside the parameters for radiation.'

So everything and everyone agreed I should have a prostatectomy. The next decision was which type and some excellent urologists in Brisbane were very helpful with this. One of the best known 'hands-on' surgeons said, 'If you can afford it, go for the robot-assisted one.' They also recommended Peter Dornan, a Brisbane physiotherapist, who runs short workshops in PC muscle strengthening to shorten the period of incontinence. I did that workshop and was pleased to find that I was already doing the exercises more intensively than recommended as a way of improving tantric sex.

So I had a radical robot-assisted prostatectomy, the benefits being a much faster recovery time, less invasive, and just as good an outcome from a treatment point of view – plus a tiny scar. My private health fund covered a good part of the huge expense. The operation went well and the urologist said the dissections afterwards indicated a 'quite aggressive' cancer. Recovery was very quick – the catheter was out in ten days and mild incontinence lasted six weeks.

I had been having erection difficulties for some years before the operation (not that uncommon in men of 60 and 70). After the operation I was referred to yet another urologist who specialised in rehabilitating erection capability post prostatectomy. He said it was important to have at least two erections a week to keep the system working and this was achieved by using penile injections – which I had been using before the operation but much less frequently. Twice a week proved too much for my battered old dick and it became scarred and misshapen. He said I had 'come to the end of the road' and all that was left was a penile implant. The final indignity!

Up till this point it hadn't made much difference whether I was gay or straight. Now I found that none of the urologists seemed interested in talking about gay sex – not that I pushed it very much. One of them said the penile implant 'will look and feel the same', which proved to be incorrect.

The other thing is that I had enormous trouble finding anyone who had a penile implant. There are 30,000 in Australia but I couldn't find one of them – straight or gay, till I finally stumbled upon John in a local support group, who very kindly spent an hour on the phone and encouraged me to go ahead.

I had already lost 1.5 inches of dick in the prostatectomy – I don't know where it went but I imagined it sliding around the floor of the surgery. I'm not sure if size is as important to a straight man as is it to a gay man but it was certainly important to me and, of course, I knew I would never ejaculate again.

The operation was very easy – it's all done through a tiny slit over the pubic bone. Somehow they manage to insert a reservoir into the abdomen, the tubes into the penis and a pump into the scrotum and then link it all up. It really is quite miraculous. The worst part of the operation was having the urologist bring in a lady doctor and they unwrapped my bruised and battered erection and he showed her how it was pumped up and down. I felt like a sideshow exhibit, but I guess I had signed a form at some stage for them to have their way with me.

Recovery was again very quick, but I went into a black period for about three months – my confidence was shattered, I lost who I was as a man and actually regretted having the prostatectomy in the first place and then the penile implant. Also, I felt very alone. I tried a couple of support groups, but couldn't talk about intimate details of my gay sex life in front of women (or even the men). I also found the groups a bit too negative. I promised myself that when all this was over, I would start up a support group for gay men with prostate cancer.

For three months, I avoided sex with anyone and avoided being seen naked. My once proud dick was a shadow of its former self in both size and angle and, worst of all, it had a droopy tip – like a Concorde taking off. I longed for the power and thrust of a Concorde (which is a bit silly, really, because at least I'm still flying and the Concorde is not). I didn't seek any help through this period but slow recovery began with some very nice encounters with empathetic men (except for the one who grabbed my balls – as gay men are likely to do. When he felt something like a piece of Lego, he went fleeing into the dark night. I quickly learned to mention the prostate cancer and its aftermath very early in an encounter – not the most romantic of seductive talk).

Two years after the prostatectomy, I have adapted to my new tool (a dick that can stay semi-hard 24/7 *is* a bit like a tool – certainly a good thing to have on a picnic). I've learned how to use it with its limitations, got used to not ejaculating and actually have very satisfying dry orgasms. And the best thing – my PSA is undetectable at the crucial two-year period and the Memorial Sloan Kettering Cancer Centre nomogram now tells me I have a 91% chance of being cancer-free in ten years time.

Yeehaa!

A gay support group has been formed and meets regularly. Contact Cancer Council Queensland for details. Other cities have them already. In the meantime, if anyone, gay or straight, needs to talk about penile implants or any other part of this journey – don't hesitate to email me at abbalean@gmail.com.

We don't have to be alone on this journey!

Three Days in Hell, Too Young!

Stephen Desmond

I was diagnosed in 2013 at 51, which I thought was too young.

I started having a flow problem in the morning (not very strong), November 2012. After two weeks, I decided to get it checked – glad I did. The GP conducted a DRE exam. He thought my prostate was a little large and said it could be an infection or maybe prostate cancer but probably not the latter given my age so I had a PSA test and he ordered an MRI scan.

PSA test came back at 3.2; MRI scan on prostate, negative.

GP said to wait three months and then we could check again.

Three months later, the PSA test came back at 3.1.

GP said wait another three months and we will check again. I said if the PSA reading comes back high what happens then? He said he would refer me to a urologist.

I said give me a referral now so I can book the appointment as specialists always have a long waiting list. If I had cancer I wanted it treated as soon as possible. My GP gave me two names on a piece of paper. I just liked the name of the first on the list so I booked with him.

Three months later my PSA came back at 4, so off to the urologist. (I did find out that my PSA was 1.5 at the age of 45, but was told by the doc at the time that all was okay. I have since found this may not have been correct and should have had a PSA test done every year.)

Glad I picked the urologist I did; he was fantastic not only with me, but with my wife. Fully explained everything and every process.

May 2014 the urologist performed a biopsy, where he took 16 samples out of my prostate and sent them away for pathology testing – not painful at all.

One week later, the results were in and, at that appointment, I was told I had cancer and that 4 out of 16 samples came back positive. He explained my Gleason Score, etc. Luckily I had my wife with me because I did not take anything in after the cancer verdict. I was classed low risk and asked how I wanted to treat it from there. The urologist went through some options.

My answer? 'Just take it out!'

I could not stand the fact I had cancer growing in me. It had to come out.

My wife and I went and had a coffee and cried a little; then I went back to work thinking I could handle it. I was wrong and broke down.

I then went on the net trying to get all the info I could over the next two weeks. Bad idea. This just overloaded me with too much info (some of it wrong) and, in the third week, I lost it completely. I then decided to talk about it with friends and family and found the PCFA website while searching the net (yes, continuing to look for info). I found the support group, rang the number and spoke with the chairperson of my local support group for 30 minutes, even though he was on holidays with his wife.

I was booked in to have a nerve-sparing radical prostatectomy on 13 August 2013, three months after deciding to have it out.

I attended the support group for the three months leading up to my operation; work was a great support with this.

I did my Kegel exercises – pelvic floor exercises, which consist of repeatedly contracting and relaxing the muscles that form part of the pelvic floor – religiously for those three months and still do them today (12 months later). These were explained to me by a continence nurse as part of the pre-operation procedure. You can do these standing up or sitting down so I do them every time I get in the car to drive. It has now become automatic.

My surgeon did a great job. The operation took six hours and went well. The three or so days in hospital recovering, not so well. I call it 'Three Days in Hell'. It was three days of vomiting, butt pain (due to the way I had to lay in the bed), no sleep, and naked patients in the middle of the night in the hospital room. The hospital stay is a story on its own.

Today, 12 months on, I have fully recovered. I have full continence control and sexual function is back to as normal as it can get, I think.

I have had three six-monthly PSA checks since and they have been .02, .03 and back to .02. Urologist said this is normal and okay.

I don't class myself as cured, as I have heard it can come back at any time – even 17 years later, so I live with this in the back of my mind every day.

My outlook on life, though, has changed. I don't worry about the small things anymore, like the kids not cleaning up their room, etc. I am just thankful that I have an absolutely wonderful family and great friends and I can enjoy being with them.

I have also realised how fast my life is passing. I used to think to myself, *I will do that later*, or think, *I'm only 30* and then, *I'm only 40; there's plenty of time to do things yet*. I know now that if you don't do things straight away and set goals, etc., you may never realise your dreams.

One of my dreams was to be in media somewhere making movies. So I made a phone call (which I would not have had the courage to do before) to a media company that produce a TV show and volunteered. It was one of the best decisions I have made, as I now have some great new friends, and am on my way. I am learning to edit, produce and film.

I also wanted to get the message out to people about prostate cancer and early detection. So I trained and qualified as a PCFA ambassador. I now do talks to spread the word about prostate cancer. One of my ambitions is to talk to young people coming out of high school to just let them know what a prostate is, what it does, find out their family history and to ensure they get checked at 40 or 50 years old. I did my first one of these at my own high school and it was received very well.

I am now 53 and, with the great support of my wife and three kids, I'm doing extremely well.

I wish to thank the people of Busybird for allowing me to share my story and wish people out there reading this the very best with their journey.

Radiation Blues

Dermot Dorgan

I used to be as healthy as anyone you'd see
but then one day my PSA was not what it should be.
The doctors took my prostate out, I thought that was the
answer,
but sad to say, to my dismay, I still had bloody cancer.
And now, I know I've got the prostate cancer radiation blues.
Oh, yes, it's so. I've got those scary-sounding, pressure-
mounting,
Geiger-counting, radiation blues.

I was perplexed. I said, 'What next?' The doctor said,
'There's ways
of treating prostate cancer with external beam x-rays.
We have to call them 'x' rays, 'cos we don't know what
they are,
but have no concern, you won't get burned, you'll just be
slightly charred.'
And now, I know I've got the prostate cancer radiation blues.
Oh, yes, it's so. I've got those ionising, sterilising,
traumatising, radiation blues.

The doctor said, 'I'm sure you've read of certain side-effects,
which as a radiation patient, you may well expect.

Your skin may start to dry out, so each day you'll need to oil it,
and for God's sake, long as you're awake, stay near a
vacant toilet.'
And now, I know I've got the prostate cancer radiation blues.
Oh, yes, it's so. I've got those stress-inducing, hair-reducing,
bowel-loosening, radiation blues.

'You'll find a way,' the doctors say, 'of dealing with fatigue.
You've felt tired before, but now you're in the major
league.
Your treatment gets priority – so put off some things till later,
'til your treatment ends, your new best friend's a Linear
Accelerator.'
And now, I know I've got the prostate cancer radiation blues.
Oh, yes, it's so. I've got those life-adjusting, doctor-trusting,
bladder-busting, radiation blues.

Oh, yes, it's so. I've got those oft-repeating, tumour-treating,
cancer beating, radiation blues.

Jousting with Authority

Ean McArthur

Associate Professor Declan Murphy recounts that before about 1990 there was often a depressing future for many prostate cancer patients. Until the Prostate Specific Antigen (PSA) blood test became available, most prostate cancers were diagnosed at an advanced stage and these cancers were incurable, with a five-year survival rate of less than 60%. To add to the patient's misery, the main treatment was castration. This entailed simply cutting off the man's testicles and thus stopping the testosterone supply, which stimulated prostate cancer growth. This was not really a cure, but only a temporary relief measure before an eventual painful death from metastatic bone cancer, with a fairly ordinary quality of life in the meantime.

I was employed by CSIRO for over 30 years, latterly as a Senior Technical Officer Grade 2, so I have some acquaintance with scientific matters. My private research revealed that until 1994 well over 1,000 Australian men per year underwent this drastic treatment of castration, although this was rarely talked about in polite society. Even as late as 2012, although many more advanced treatments were available and cancers were being detected earlier, the number of castrations was still well over 120 per year. Overseas numbers for prostate cancer castrations are staggering, often running into thousands per year, mainly because castration is a 'once off' treatment and far cheaper than the alternative of chemical implants, and tablets, which also suppress the testosterone level. Thus, for instance, there were 6,246 cases in the USA in 2005. The numbers for some less-developed countries are also in the thousands and a Swedish study had a cohort of 17,000 Swedish men who had been castrated as a treatment for prostate cancer.

I once met an old man at an Aging Well Expo who confided to me, 'Well, actually, I've lost my nuts. My doctor used to line us up six at a time and do us all in the one day.'

I said, 'Shit, he must have worked on a sheep station once.'

What a sad day's work that would be, but still it was better than pushing up the daisies before your time.

I myself joined this unhappy band in 1999, although in my case it was not advanced prostate cancer but localised cancer, picking the wrong urologist and getting rushed into treatment. Some people, like me, are just born stupid. As an old German saying goes, 'We get too soon old and too late smart.'

There is a wide selection of prostate cancer treatments available today and there is vastly more patient information and support available than there was 10 to 15 years back. This is to the great credit of the medical profession and the Prostate Cancer Foundation of Australia. Public awareness about prostate cancer has exploded over the last ten years and it is now common for men to make the most extensive enquiries before deciding on a treatment. I certainly don't knock this approach for it is far better to be sure than sorry. The underlying problem with any Androgen Deprivation Treatment (ADT) - castration or chemical - as applied to advanced prostate cancer, is that the cancer eventually becomes castrate resistant (less controllable) and the cancer then progresses throughout the body. There is also the problem of side-effects, which include osteoporosis, anemia, muscle wastage, hot flushes, impotence, depression and cognitive impairment. Osteoporosis can be overcome by various medications and exercises. The bone density can be increased back to normal levels in this way, and this definitely happened in my case, by means of testosterone and Actonel medications. For most patients, testosterone augmentation is definitely inadvisable, but in my case we were only restoring the testosterone level to the lower side of normal range to counter the side-effects. Early on when I asked a doctor about using testosterone, his reply was quite blunt: 'Do you want to end up as a little jar of ashes on the mantelpiece?' Very few doctors would prescribe testosterone where prostate cancer was involved. After all, they are aiming to suppress the testosterone, not enhance it.

Regarding impotence and low libido, well, you can get used to it after a time, but in the real world, the triple whammy of castration, radiation and advanced age pegs one back to somewhere near zero. Erectile Dysfunction treatments may be helpful for some patients. The incidence of erectile dysfunction may tend to be underestimated by the medical profession, but patients tell a different story.

Some support groups have amassed huge libraries of books on prostate cancer. Many of these books are absolute rubbish, some promoting ridiculous alternative treatments. Any book with the words 'prostate cancer' in the title will most likely sell by the thousands regardless of merit, and some celebrities like to tell the world about their 'courageous' battle with prostate cancer. Let's face it, there is a market out there. There are, of course, many excellent technical books and DVDs, particularly by leading Australian urologists and The Prostate Cancer Foundation of Australia (PCFA).

I was diagnosed with localised prostate cancer in 1999 (with a PSA of 7.8 and a Gleason score 5 or 6). The urologist's very brief summary of possible treatments went as follows: 'Radiation is no good for you because it has gotten into your bones.' He then proposed orchidectomy (castration) saying, 'Chemical treatment will have the same effect on impotency and has cardiac risks.' Upon hearing 'it has gotten into your bones,' which turned out to be incorrect, I thought that this meant that the cancer had spread and the outlook was grim. I have had a life-long weakness for complying with those in authority, be it my mother, my teacher, my NCO, or my doctor, so I reluctantly agreed with his recommendation. Far from being a cure, my troubles were just starting. After a year, my PSA was doubling every few months and I needed seven weeks of radiation treatment, which virtually stopped the cancer but produced additional side-effects as well.

I was never in the least happy with being castrated. When I became depressed after the operation, I joined a prostate cancer support group and learned that none of these chaps had had this treatment, which they regarded as rare, antiquated and unusual. Mind you, two of them had been offered this same treatment by the very same doctor, but had wisely made for the door and never went back again.

At my first support group Christmas party, I was called up to the front and given a nicely wrapped present, which I was urged to open and display then and there. With some reluctance and suspicion, I found it contained two peeled hard-boiled eggs. I was grateful that it was not testicles sourced from the local slaughter house. Some people love these rough little jokes; others just give a sickly grin.

My castration was always at the back of my mind and, after about eight years, I decided to make a complaint (technically termed a notification) to the Medical Practitioners Board of Victoria (MPB). The matter was well outside the limitation of actions period of three years for a civil action in the courts, so there could be no money in it for me, just a thirst for justice. The time limitation did not apply to the MPB action but the MPB was a tough nut to crack – as one would expect with a self-regulated body – and I was advised by a well-informed friend that a win was unlikely. An academic study of MPB complaints in the financial year 2004–2005 recorded 690 complaints, not all by patients. Of these complaints, 7% resulted in adverse findings, including 5% who received only cautions. In my own case, the doctor's defence (produced after consulting his Medical Defence Association) was that he did not remember me as a patient, nor did he remember operating on me. All his relevant patient records no longer existed but he certainly would have explained everything about the range of treatments possible, and he would have acted in accordance within the highest professional standards.

The process ran for three years and had two appeals before there was a finding of 'unprofessional conduct' and a formal reprimand for my dear old surgeon. Unfortunately, he had retired from practice many years before, so it did not have an impact on him other than a dent in his pride. Was the process worth it for me? Yes, it most definitely was.

After this little battle, I moved on to publicising the situation and pressing for the abolishment or severe restriction of this outmoded treatment. This may sound like a tall order, but after all, this treatment had already been supplanted 1,000 to 1 by chemical castration. Chemical castration does the same job but has the great advantage that it allows intermittent treatment, which postpones the onset of castrate-resistant prostate cancer – a very important advantage indeed. In addition, chemical castration allows intermittent relief from the drastic side-effects, which is no small thing. Castration is, of course, irreversible – you can't sew the bastards back on!

My *crusade* sounded logical enough to me, but in an age of massive public comment it was hard to get a word in edgewise, be it letters to the editor, letters to politicians, or whatever. As an 80-year-old, I had no experience of these new-fangled things like Twitter or Facebook or webpages and, in fact, I had a strong distaste for them, as they seem to attract a heap of garbage. I was also rather a nervous and ineffectual public speaker and I found that many people in power were resistant to any suggestions coming from the lower deck. I tried writing to *The Age*, my local State Member and the State Minister for Health and so on, but there was never the ghost of a reply. I decided not to touch the tabloid press.

A charity lobbyist once told me that the reality was that every politician – and particularly ministers – received around 1,000 letters a day. Their office would sort out a dozen or so letters for attention and reply – mostly letters that could cause them grief and pain or were in the public eye. The rest would be put on the backburner and never saw the light of day. I certainly did not have the gift of being an effective lobbyist. Perhaps the real secret would be to employ a spin doctor, but those boys can really charge like wounded bulls.

I had written to my Federal Member, The Hon Mark Dreyfus, QC. MP and, after a reminder, his office sprang into action and forwarded my letter to the Minister for Health, for which I was grateful. In the meantime, I explored sending a petition to Parliament. Although these petitions normally have numerous signatures, this is not essential as long as the petition is respectful and complies with the guidelines. I felt that a lone petition, properly worded, would have as much impact as one main petitioner and a flock of sheep. Thus the Petition was as follows:

> This petition of an 81-year-old survivor of prostate cancer and castration, draws to the attention of the House the continuing use of the outmoded and unnecessary procedure of surgical castration as a treatment for prostate cancer and the severe physical and emotional harms resulting there from.
>
> We therefore ask the House to enquire into and take such action as may lead to the abolition of this procedure within Australia.

This petition was presented formally in the House of Representatives on 11 February 2013 and was then referred to the Minister for Health for action.

Actually, in a separate letter to the Health Minister, I modified my request to 'abolish or severely restrict the use of this treatment.' Alas, alas, it was not going to be that easy, but did I really expect a walkover? Rather than considering and comparing the intrinsic clinical merits of the two alternatives of surgical castration and chemical castration, the reply revolved around the individual patient's theoretical right to choose his preferred type of hormone deprivation treatment, as specified in the Clinical Guidelines. This stunned me as, statistically, the actual patient preference in practice was about 1,000 to 1 against surgical castration. If you stopped any man in the street and asked him whether he would like to be castrated, you are absolutely certain to get no takers and you would definitely get some rude replies into the bargain. The typical construction of these clinical guidelines ran along the lines that the eminent committee (including numerous professors) would review all the current research and practice on a particular treatment at great length and then conclude that there was insufficient evidence available to make a definite recommendation at that time. This is exactly what happened in this case. To fasten onto this one clause, which was interpreted as upholding the holy supremacy of patient preference, was unbelievable to me. Surely the focus should have been on the comparative clinical merits of these two treatments, including the numbers involved, and the historical picture, and not on this isolated theme of patient preference, which seemed to me to be a red herring and a brush-off.

'I've met a number of men who are very thankful that they have had an orchidectomy rather than the chemical form of hormone therapy with all its possible side-effects and I've met many men that regret following the chemical castration solution because of the very severe side-effects they have suffered. In any of these decisions it is clear to me that quality of life issues need to be fully considered before taking a particular option.'

As far as I am concerned this is still only round one of the debate.

Breaking the rule that you never present the other side of the story in an adversarial situation, there are, in fact, some very few instances where urologists consider surgical castration may be the better option. These cases are when there is advanced prostate cancer with considerable bone metastases and pain, and this is when surgical castration will give much faster relief. This should be seen in the context that there were about 128 cases of surgical castration for prostate cancer in 2012 compared with over 60,000 prescriptions for

Zoladex, the most common anti-androgen medication, which costs something like $1,200 a shot.

The other side of the coin is that there must be many cases like mine where the patients had only localised prostate cancer but were still castrated by certain surgeons of the old school, who stuck to the old ways and did not advance with the times.

Medicare has very good statistics dating from 1994 when their records started and I have accessed many of these. Castrations in Australia have decreased by about 90% over a 20-year period. The numbers vary remarkably between states, being high in Queensland and practically zero in ACT and NT.

I was secretary of a Prostate Cancer Support Group for about 11 years and, over this period, 10 or more of our brave chaps lost their fight against the disease. They came along to the group until near the very end, seeking a grain of comfort from fellow members. We had a system whereby after the formal business, we went around the circle and each member reported on their own medical condition and progress. The individual reports varied. Some chaps expanded on quite a bit of medical detail, some strayed into weird alternative treatments, and some gave us a bit of humour and an insight into their background. Some of these brave chaps came along with a sheaf of notes to update us on their last losing battle and tell us that this would be their last appearance. Woman's breast cancer support groups seem to operate on a quite different level, and the women really do things so much better. They ditch some of the formal business and are more into friendship, compassion and empathy, whereas we stoic and reserved old fellows tend to treat meetings more like a business meeting.

There was a doctor who regularly attended our support group incognito, and who later died of advanced prostate cancer himself. He was a nice, unassuming chap and he must have chuckled as he sat up the back and listened to some of our 'experts' sounding off.

Support groups provide companionship and emotional support to the members, as well as provide a great deal of information. It is preferable that patients get this information at the earliest stage before treatment is decided. I feel that some groups can get too formal and business-like, to the detriment of the emotional support side.

At this point in proceedings on 13 May 2013, my wife Rosemary died at home from a sudden heart attack after 54 years of marriage. She was a wonderful companion, an ex-teacher, a great reader and a keen family history researcher. She quietly disapproved of my little jousts with authority, bless her! She was a keen gardener, so now I have inherited the responsibility of tending the garden, looking after our cat and feeding the lorikeets and possums. We had the funeral service at the little local church so that some of the locals could walk to the service.

We never expect things like this, do we?

My Prostate Cancer as an Adventure, Not a Journey!

Roger Northam

Since my diagnosis three years ago, whenever the subject of prostate cancer arises – which is frequently – it seems that the conversation heads automatically in a negative direction. Sadly, for many men, there is good reason for negativity, and I was initially amongst that group.

My regular blood tests showed a rising PSA at the age of 65, which is not uncommon, but a DRE (also known as a finger up your rear end!) suggested that it was probably worth taking the next step – a biopsy. At the time, I thought this was just about the worst day of my life. That is until I received the results a couple of days after, along with the dreaded words, 'Sorry, but the biopsy showed a positive result. You have prostate cancer.'

For most of us, life just rolls along with only the occasional blip. I had constantly read about the 'Big C', as it is described by many, but of course that was for others – not *me*.

Here, suddenly, it was *me*. I had cancer.

I walked out of the surgery with my wife, totally stunned. All I could think was, *Why me?* My next response was to get things in order. Funny how the brain responds to pressure.

But, if I had thought that I had already experienced the worst day of my life, more was to come. The urologist assured me there was no rush and that I needed to consider and choose between three options: wait and watch, have a radical prostatectomy (have a what? Note how a lot of new words had come into my life!), or do nothing (sort of 'it may go away').

I'm an action man. So, if I had this 'thing' growing inside me, I had to get rid of it. I found out what a prostatectomy was and decided that would be my course.

How I wish I had gone to a local support group and spoken to those who had had actual experience with all this! I probably wouldn't have made a different decision, but I would have been better informed.

My operation was deemed successful, but I was warned that I would have to stay free of cancer for five years before I was really in the clear. Only a few months later I had a positive PSA reading. It was low, but sufficient that I was advised to have radiation treatment. Wow – another new term I had to learn about!

I was as scared as hell when I went for my first treatment, but I met some truly wonderful, caring people. After 36 treatments (read: two months), I had made some new friends in the radiation centre whom I would not have met without my cancer. No, it may not have been an ideal way to make friends, but in spite of the seriousness of my predicament, I found myself actually having a bit of fun along the way.

I was strongly drawn to the idea of assisting other men in a similar position, and I became an active member of my local support group. Soon after, I joined the Victorian PCFA Chapter. I began meeting all sorts of interesting people and got involved in things that I would never have done were it not for my prostate cancer.

This may sound a little weird, but, at the age of 69, I have to say that the last three years have been exciting. Through mixing with people with a similar problem I have made some great friends. I have also been able to see that, while cancer is serious, it is possible to stay positive and maintain hope about the future when you share experiences with other people in a similar position and undertake the right treatment. Recently, I went to New Zealand for a motorcycle championship with a new support group friend. I had lost sight of my love of motorbikes over the years, and as I stood there watching the racing, I reflected that I had my prostate cancer to thank for bringing it back to me. In fact, I could tell of many similar, smaller examples of such discoveries or rediscoveries.

My life has definitely become more of an adventure and less of a straightforward journey. What I now see is that, although it has been sad, my prostate cancer has helped me to understand that we are all terminal. We don't know how long we'll be here, and I feel lucky to have this early warning call that I am ageing. I am in pretty good health for my age, and I have a loving family and fabulous grandchildren. I have learned to get on with life and enjoy what I have left, and I have learned to trust my specialists.

When the time comes, I am going to look back and say, loudly, my head held high, 'Wow, how good was that! Thanks to my prostate cancer, I have had a nice little adventure to wrap up my time in this world. What a ride it's been!'

Dance, Jimmy, Dance

Gavin Haberfield

Dance, Jimmy, you wicked boy,
Comes the news, no room for joy.
My manhood vandalised, my loss acute,
and you dance your dance, hidden and mute.
All fear and bluff to plan the fight,
so I must wait to measure this night.
Loved ones told, it needs to sink in,
while you dance your dance without any sin.

Gleason has spoken and so it shall be,
the lot has to go so that I can pee.
But what else to lose? There's so much more,
so much remains for me in store.
Jimmy, dance your dance and carve your path,
I plan to be rid of you before the half.
While robots strike and remove the rotten,
you dance a dance that cannot be forgotten.

I want me rid of thee dancer, Jim,
You are making time utterly miserably grim.

Welcome news that the stage is early,
this thing that shades everything so surely.
Early or not, it does not change the sum,
and no lesser the task ahead to come.
No rush, be calm, take time to study,
make experts and the learned your very best buddy.
Make a choice but be sure to choose no fluke;
a surgical strike or take a nuke.

The choice is known, what a relief.
A surgeon's knife for this hideous thief.
So, now the days pass as I wait for my time,
getting checkups from where the sun don't shine.
What's really in store, I really don't know,
But the sooner it is here, the better the show.
So dance your dance, Jimmy, and care not a pittance,
'cos very soon I'll celebrate your good riddance.

The Kid

Danielle de Valera

'Life's funny,' my neighbour, Ron, said to me one day when we were on our second cup of coffee. 'When the oncologist told me I had cancer, I was like, *Whoa! What are we going to do about it?* The oncologist told me there was nothing we could do. He was adamant. I asked him how much time I had and he told me maybe five months. The next thing I remember is sitting on the sofa in the lounge room. The Kid was out, the clock said 4.00 pm. Somewhere along the way, I'd lost three hours, and now, in five months or so, I was going to lose my life. Want another Scotch Finger?'

'Ta.' It was comforting to know the ocean was still there, still roaring for me. It would still be there when I needed it.

'Well,' said Ron, 'I poured myself a stiff bourbon and sat there. At first, I was angry. Why me? What had I ever done that was so wrong?' Ron passed me the Scotch Fingers. 'Then, after a while, something changed in me and I thought, *Well, if that's how it is, that's how it is. Might as well accept it.* So there I sat, resigning myself to the inevitable. The Kid was out raging somewhere – probably riding his trail bike around the nature reserve and ripping up the dunes. He was sixteen then, a hard kid to raise.

'At five o'clock, I began planning my funeral. I'd just picked out the pallbearers when, out of the blue, it hit me.' Ron thumped himself on the chest. 'IF I DIE, WHO'S GONNA LOOK AFTER THE KID?

'My ex, she'd remarried, and the new man and The Kid didn't get on. Well, I thought, the ex is out, even though she's his mother. Who else was there? I had no brothers, no sisters. My father was 82; he couldn't do it. Besides, he'd remarried – why is everyone remarrying these days? If you met someone else now Harry's gone, would you marry them?'

'Don't think so,' I said through a mouthful of Scotch Fingers.

''Course you wouldn't. Anyway, Dad's new wife didn't want him to have anything to do with us, apart from a card at Christmas. The Kid couldn't go there. What to do?

'And that's when I decided I couldn't die after all. Just when I was getting used to the idea and thinking what music I'd like at the service. No one else was going to look after that kid. They'd toss him into foster care and he'd end up in jail. Can't let that happen, I thought. He might be a bastard, but he's my kid and he needs me.

'So I had another drink and pulled myself together. By the time I heard The Kid's bike coming down the road, I had the water on for the spaghetti and was frying up the mince for the sauce – he loves spaghetti bol', it's his favourite.

'And that's it, really.' Ron spread out his hands. 'All that was six years ago, the oncologist can't believe it! I swear, I was ready to let them take me until I remembered The Kid. Funny how life works out, isn't it?'

He gave me a hug at the door. 'Have a good one.' And when I reached the road, instead of turning right to the ocean, I turned left for home.

Parkes on Prostate

Richard Parkes

Diagnosis

'Hey, Doc, the waterworks are not working as well as they used to.'

'Well, we have been following your PSA blood tests, but two is not excessive. The finger test says your prostate is enlarged, but nothing seems unusual.'

This is the start of a journey you wish you were not taking!

The PSA goes to 2.5 and there are still issues with the waterworks – dribbling, wanting to go more often, and being difficult to control. The doctor sends me to a urologist. He puts me on Flowmaxtra, which 'should improve your flow'. There's not much improvement, though, and the PSA moves up to 3.5.

The next move is to look up my 'old man' and take pictures of what is going on. For me, this is in January 2009. The result is, 'Hey Rick, you have an enlarged prostate, which is blocking your bladder, and there is some scarring in the bladder.'

I ask the doctor what this means.

He tells me that he is trying to manage my problem with Flowmaxtra, but he thinks there is a need to improve the flow through surgery; this is called a TURP – transurethral resection of the prostate. But it may be time to do a biopsy; this will tell if there are early stages of cancer. If not, he can carry on with a TURP.

'Hey, what if it's cancer?'

'It may mean radical surgery – in other words, remove the prostate.' This is February 2009 and I am due in Nepal for a trek to Everest Base Camp.

We decide to wait until I return in April. After a successful trek in Nepal, another PSA is carried out and indicates a reading of five – not a good sign after 15 years of tracking. Two major jumps in a short period, but still not considered excessive. The decision is made for a biopsy in July, after a trip to Thailand. July 17th, I go into Wesley for a biopsy. They knock me out, take 18 strips off my prostate for testing, and take more photos. This proves to be a bad day; I have money stolen from my wallet during the biopsy, and then the news comes that I have the early stages of prostate cancer.

'Who – me? Shit.' The next step is to have a bone scan. Now, this worries me; does it mean it may have spread? So, back again to the Wesley on the 22nd for a bone scan. Thank God that is clear.

On 28th July, Sue and I see the specialist. It appears I have early stages – what they call T1 – which indicates it is confined to the prostate, and a Gleason score of seven (3+4). A score of two to five indicates the cancer is relatively slow-growing and probably not very aggressive. A score from five to seven indicates the cancer is faster growing and moderately aggressive. A score of eight or higher indicates an aggressive cancer.

Then, the doc indicates a node on my prostate, which is causing the blockage.

What next?

Decision Time

There appears to be three approaches: watch and wait, surgery (remove the bloody thing), or radiation therapy.

Watch and wait does not appear to be an option, as the node is blocking my bladder and that will not improve. As I have an early warning, let's do something.

After receiving the news of my cancer, I begin researching. My research is leaning me towards surgery, and I have read of the success of robotic surgery, which improves the chances of less damage to critical nerves that control your ability for erections and future void control (controlling incontinency). This is not a simple issue, and there are many factors to consider.

A good friend, Richard, is due to have surgery on 29th July. He had been in Brisbane earlier that month, before the biopsy. We had had a good chat about the options and his decision-making.

My Saturday walking group also had a number of inflicted gentlemen – all had surgery. When I tell one of my walking friends, Terry, of the diagnosis, he says he knows a sports physiotherapist who had his prostate removed many years ago and is now a leader of the local Brisbane support group. He has written a book and specialises in exercises for incontinence. I give him a ring and have a chat; he was operated on 13 years ago and found that there was no support, becoming depressed in regards to incontinence and erectile dysfunction. This drove him to develop a support group, and as a physiotherapist he understands the importance of pelvic floor exercise to help reduce the problem of incontinence – before and after the operation. My specialist also referred me to Peter regarding the importance of these exercises.

Within a week of my diagnoses, I have a session with Peter and another four guys, all very nervous of the future and all with diagnoses of cancer. We are told of Peter's experience and instructed in pelvic floor exercises, which are about the actions of 'stopping yourself peeing', 'pretending to stop a fart' and 'imagining getting away from a red hot poker between your anus and scrotum'. This is all at the same time. I assure you, it's not easy, and especially as you cannot see the muscles you are working on.

Once these exercises are mastered, they should be carried out in conjunction with the 'crunch exercise' and 'bicycle crunch', plus other activities, such as walking, cycling and jogging.

During the week I also go to my first support group meeting, which is targeted at the more advanced forms of prostate cancer. The main speaker is Professor Paul Mainwaring, who talks about new developments and therapies for treatment of advanced prostate cancer. I guess many of the group have not been as lucky as myself with early detection. It appears that much of the treatment is still very experimental, but I guess, if life is being shortened, you will try anything. It was not the greatest night, but it made me realise the options available, and that, in the end, you have to make the final decision yourself.

Meanwhile, Sue and I decide to push on with our world trip before making the final decision on what action to take. It is decided that I should see the urologist Dr X – who is experienced with robotic surgery – on my return. This is booked in for 25th September, and a provisional robotic surgery booking for 18th November. I am 70% certain that this is going to be my course of action.

In July, we head off for the US, the UK, France, Singapore, and then back to Brisbane. It is a great trip, and I feel fit and well and a bit of a fraud with this cancer thing niggling away inside. I decide to be quite open about the problem, as I want my friends and family to know that it is something that I am going to defeat.

The 25th of September looms, and Sue and I head off to an appointment with Dr X. He is an upfront, capable sort of fellow who believes that the right approach for me is surgery, especially as I am fit and should have a good twenty years ahead of me. The warnings of incontinence and erectile problems are confirmed. The potential issues in this area should stand a better chance with robotic surgery. Dr X has performed 80 operations using the Da Vinci machine, and 2,000 old-fashioned ops.

So at the moment of 5 October 2009, the decision is to remove the prostate on the morning of the 18th November. Meanwhile, I am working hard on pelvic muscles and my general fitness. In myself, I feel good, and of course the doubts of radical surgery start niggling in your mind, so it is important to keep reading and asking questions all the time to confirm your decision-making. I make an appointment with my GP to talk it through and maybe get another PSA check. I also speak to Richard in WA, who had the operation nine weeks ago. He is feeling pretty good and his PSA is zero. His incontinence is on the mend, although it is too early to tell on the erection front!

The startling thing is that the media seems full of stories on prostate cancer and one tends to get bombarded with information. But, when it comes down to it, it remains *my decision*.

I see my GP on Friday and we have a positive conversation and she agrees with my approach. We discuss Dr X; she has heard good reports, so I am now very positive and will concentrate on getting as fit as I can, plus build up my pelvic muscles.

Pre-Operation Period

The guys at the walking group all show interest, so this becomes a positive defacto support group.

During the week (9.10.2009), a research group from the Cancer Council *ProsCan* makes contact. This is a new program of research to find better ways to assist men with prostate cancer and their partners. It appears prostate cancer is the current flavour. Charlene rings me and will meet Sue and myself next Wednesday. We will take as much help as we can get, and maybe help others in the future.

Charlene is part of a research group *ProsCan for Couples*, made up of Cancer Council and Griffith University and is all about developing an educational support program for men with prostate cancer and their partners to assist them in adjusting to the diagnosis of prostate cancer and the outcomes of treatment, particularly sexual changes.

We meet on Wednesday; Charlene gives us the lowdown and we both fill out questionnaires. We have also been allocated a kind of mentor – a nurse – who will discuss our progress before and after.

After the op, we will be bombarded with questionnaires over the next twelve months to see how our lives have changed – mainly our sex life.

On Friday, I receive a big package from *ProsCan* research – booklets for Sue and myself to take us through the trials and tribulations and frustrations of the coming months.

The exercises continue and the general fitness regime is increased. A month to 'P-day'.

It is now 29th October. The fitness regime continues, and I believe I have the hang of pelvic exercises, though it's hard to tell as it's all inside. (I can lift my balls, and have movement around my scrotum, using the mirror!) So, it's starting to happen, and I am up to 140 bicycling crunches to strengthen my stomach area.

Today I receive a parcel from Queensland University, regarding Bio Resource, as I am donating my prostate to the tissue bank. Another long form to fill out, asking some eighty questions about myself, including my state of baldness, the origins of my family, sex life, etc. I guess trying to analyse trends may help find the origins of the cancer and identify who is likely to be susceptible.

Today Sylvia, my contact nurse from *ProsCan*, was on the phone, and we had a good 40-minute chat about expectations before and after the op, trying to understand our stress levels and talking through any uncertainties. My major one is how soon can I get back to my usual activity level?

It is a difficult time, especially when one receives the November issue of *Prostate Cancer News* – headline: **Brachytherapy regarded as superior treatment for prostate cancer**. This comes out of two independent studies from the Prostate Cancer Foundation of Chicago and the Taussig Cancer Centre at Cleveland. Just another piece of information that adds to the doubts about the surgery option. Good survival rates, less invasive, better incontinence rates, and less chance of sexual dysfunction – up to 25%.

Who do you believe?

It's 4th November and I have a long talk with Jenny, Dr X's specialist urology nurse. We discuss the planning of the prostatectomy and the preplanning of Microlax enema – she suggested two instead of one.

She then explained that once the op, which could take five hours, was over, I would be wearing white stockings and boots to stop any blood clotting. Also, I will be fitted with a large catheter bag and have a drip in my arm. Don't be surprised if there is blood in the urine!

The next day they will fit me with a smaller bag (drink plenty of water) to reduce the chance of constipation. Constipation will cause pressure on the catheter tube and prevent flow of urine.

The day-to-day catheter bag is fitted to the leg by two tapes, rubbery side against the leg to stop slipping; the bag has a tap which you use to discharge into the toilet. Still could be blood around.

We also talked about how long the incontinence problems would occur, and this will be dependent on the nerve damage. Less likely at night when resting but will occur when carrying out activities such as lifting, getting up from bed, etc. Must not get into gym or excessive activities until Dr X gives the word. Could take up to six months to be dry but could be sooner.

Nurses at hospital will give away sample pads when you leave and after the catheter is removed. Pads are available in supermarket, but make sure they are incontinency pads (have droplets on cover, more drops the larger the pad). Men can use women's pads; the smaller ones attach to the underwear, larger ones just fit in.

If I require painkillers, ask nurses but should not use codeine-based but Tramil as codeine is an opioid and has side-effects such as urination.

Try to train bladder habits away from lots of small occurrences otherwise the brain will train itself to operate the bladder that way.

'Drink plenty of water, keep away from caffeine and alcohol.'

We talked about dry erections and orgasms (brain function, not physical), and also the potential need for help, such as Viagra, or injections. Also the possibility of urine leakage during sex. The old adage 'use it or lose it' was discussed.

The 6th of November – reached 200 bicycle crunches. I hope to reach 400 like Elle Macpherson the model, which she does every day.

The 13th of November – my 66th birthday today – and five days to go. Spoke to Richard Bingham, who is about 15 weeks post-operation and confirms a nil PSA and not experiencing incontinence. He has not recovered his sex life, but talked to a friend of his in Adelaide who also had the op; he has been given a mixed chemical which has helped his erections already.

This week paid up my $11,000 in advance to the surgeon. It is important to understand the costs, especially during this stressful time.

I also spoke with Greenslopes regarding my admission, giving MBF and Medicare numbers. I also spoke with a nurse about the details of arrival and the operation. No jewellery, plenty of books and magazines, loose clothes and keep smiling.

The 14th of November, walked Mt Cootha with the usual group. Everyone was supportive and wished me the best. Met a guy who has been on *watch and wait* for five years; he diets and takes alternative medicine to keep his PSA down, but, as one learns, the measurement of PSA is a deceptive marker.

The 17th of November, 220 bicycle crunches and we talk to Sylvia from *ProsCan*. She reinforces the possible problems after the surgery – incontinence, erectile dysfunction, how to deal with catheters. She asks about our stress levels as a number between one and ten, ten being the highest. I mark myself three, Sue four – mine about apprehension and dependence on other people regarding success, e.g. surgeons; Sue is worried about a loved one and the uncertainty.

Need to get info regarding contacts when let out of hospital if any problems (catheter).

The Operation

Well, today is 'P-Day'.

I am up early at 4.30 am for an enema, the second one in seven hours, so now all cleared out.

Sue and myself head for Greenslopes Hospital and arrive for 7.00 am admission. The paperwork starts; I give my name and date of birth a dozen times, (this makes sure they have the right person for the right operation).

Next, onto the blood-letting nurse. Before that, I change into gown, paper knickers, TED tights and paper booties; then I move onto ECG machine.

Around 7.30 am I say farewell to Sue and begin rolling towards the anesthetist ante-ward, following in a traffic jam of trollies.

My anesthetist is an Indian who calls me 'Mate' and 'Boss' and reminds me of Malaysia. He starts by sticking a drip in, ready to give me my knockout juice.

Next stop, the operating theatre and on the way see Dr X, my surgeon, and shake hands. I am all set up and the anesthetist chats to me and applies the 'magic juice'.

Post-Operation

Next, I remember is waking up in my private room, less a prostate, and with a catheter fitted out of the 'old man', a draining tube out of my stomach and a drip in my arm. As I was drifting in and out on morphine, I did not remember many of the things Sue or the nurses said. Sue claimed I was asking lots of questions and being cheeky to the nurses, but I do remember that she told me the operation went well and that Dr X got all the cancer.

Sue left at 5.00 pm and the next day had to remind me of what went on.

I then went into television mode plus dozing. All through the night I am monitored and the registrar allows me some juice and chicken broth. I have another couple of morphine doses. The pee bag is filling up well, which is a good sign, though still bloody. I do not have any real pain – just a dull ache in the stomach. I am given blood thinners and antibiotics. The registrar continues to visit and checks my pee. It was a long night and I spent some time reading until 12.00 am.

In the morning, breakfast consisted of a couple of juices and a cup of tea.

Then the procedure of taking me off the drip and the drainage tube begins (surprising how long). Had a trainee nurse, who was very nervous doing the procedure. The nurses then take off my socks and blow up leggings to ready me for a shower. I'm a bit groggy as I get out of bed and my stomach muscles feel as if they have had a round with Muhammad Ali. I shuffle to the shower carrying my pee bag. It is great to have a shower, and have to exercise great care around the 'old man' – it's a bit disconcerting having a catheter sticking out the end. I also have a shave (must keep the morale up).

Just as I am leaving the shower Dr X arrives and says they got the cancer and confirmed that the prostate was enlarged, but it went better than he thought, and I did not lose too much blood. There was a slight warning about incontinence being longer because of the large prostate – still, that is the next challenge! After the catheter is removed, I make a follow-up appointment, then a PSA check in three months.

Next, a change of pee bag to one that is attached to my leg – a little uncomfortable but just have to get used to it. Dr X suggested getting out of hospital this afternoon or next morning. I opt for next morning.

After all this activity – now mid-morning – I am offered two sandwiches and a cup of tea, which I wolf down. I am on a light diet; do not want to put too much pressure on bowel movements.

I go for a walk around the ward – not sure catheter working 100%. All these things are new?

Sue arrives at 12. It is good to see her. Nurse A comes in to give me an antibiotic jab. *Ahh!* My first pain; the vein is closing up. She continues. Bloody painful! Ten minutes later comes back with another jab to enlarge the vein. Still doing blood pressures and temperature.

Sue says goodbye at 3.30 pm – I am feeling good for one day in.

Next, a dinner for a flea arrives – a little cottage pie, carrots and potatoes.

I am having stomach pain, due to blowing up during the operation – need to keep farting to clear. At about 7.00 am another set of injections – blood thinner and dreaded antibiotic. Nurse goes slowly but still bloody painful.

At midnight, the night nurse, Mary, decides against the antibiotic jab after trying other veins on my left arm and not being successful. Little while later I have pain under the left rib-cage and Mary gives me Panadeine and a peppermint tea – the dreaded wind build-up. I eventually get to sleep.

Woke at 4.30 am with further pain in the shoulders and stomach – have a green tea. Pain slowly dissipates.

Registrar arrives and looks at my stomach-entry cuts, and gives me the all clear.

I go into shower and take off all the tapes – have a shave and put on clothes. Nurse A not very forthcoming about the discharge procedure.

Nurse A gives me my discharge papers, plus night bags for the week and an extra catheter leg bag. At this time it is important to get information regarding disposal of night bag contents and the hygiene required around the catheter and bags. I was offered very little.

Sue arrives at 10.30 am and we head for home. The car being low made the journey unpleasant; felt very tight under my testicles.

I am having a down day and not as bright as the previous day. I guess escaping the protection offered by the hospital has now gone.

Have stomach pain and would like to make a bowel movement, but not allowed to force it. Given Movicol to assist – but not working yet; also on Panamax for pain.

I stooge around for rest of the day, reading and being lazy and a bit down in the dumps.

A bit uncomfortable during the night, a headache and a need to have a bowel movement. I also fix another night bag about 2.00 am as I fill my first one. In the morning, I am uncertain; what do I do with night bags? And do we clean out the leg bag? A little bit of information that would have been useful from the hospital!

I decide to ring Dr X's rooms and guess what? No one available until Monday; *if there is an emergency go to your local hospital* – a bit different than the Registrar's information. Confucius says, 'Make sure you get an actual number before leaving the hospital.'

We then make contact with our prostate network and Meron, an ex-nurse friend, agrees we cut the night bags and dispose of urine and that the leg bag is for the duration. Cannot be cleaned. It is important not to get downhearted, especially with the catheter, and try to be positive, reminding oneself that the cancer has been removed.

Eureka! Saturday, 21st November, 9.00 am, I have a bowel movement. It's amazing what makes you happy.

Over the last three days managed to get a couple of one-kilometre walks in the garden; the pool's 25 metres so I target 40 lengths. I have had my ups and downs in these days and find different parts of the body play up. Yesterday, the 'old fellow' had a dull ache all day and the base where it meets the testicles was painful. It may have been caused by putting on tighter underwear. This was done because I thought it would keep the catheter and old fellow in place. Though not sure as took them off at night, but still woke up with pain at night in those areas and had to take painkillers.

This morning all appears okay. Another pain is from an entry scar on my left side below the ribs, which has been roughly sewn up.

Over these few days I have had challenges around night pee bags, changes of appointments for extraction of catheter and claiming for cost recovery. I am surprised at the scale of charges from Dr X – $4,500 above the schedule fee, and only get $376 from MBF towards that. What is private insurance about?

Wednesday, 25th November, had another rough night; pain seems to return to scrotum and penis area, aggravated by the catheter.

The catheter removal has been confirmed for Sunday. *Great!*

Felt great during the day – walked one kilometre. Dr X phoned and was asking how I was and gave me the result of the biopsy of the removed prostate; confirmed did contain cancer, a pT2c with Gleason score of seven and the marginal status was focal positivity, and that there was a slight chance it may have moved on, but his view was positive and doubted it had. I need to understand how that can be determined. My next appointment will be 29th December.

Friday 28th November, I am improving; walked two kilometres over the day and did not get tired. Sleeping far better at night. I am very appreciative of the concern and good wishes of all my friends across the world. It means a lot at this time.

Catheter Removal

Sunday, we are up early for an 8.30 am appointment at Greenslopes. We arrive and go through reception and, as the Urology Ward has no beds. We end up in Ward 35, the surgical ward.

This ward does not have experienced urology nurses so have to explain about my operation and the incontinence effects – the void and retain procedure are different than the norm.

The nurse deflates the balloon holding the catheter in the bladder by using a syringe into the spare tube (red end). Then pulls the catheter. This was bloody painful as it slid out, but did not last long.

At last, free of the bloody catheter!

Now it's time to drink plenty of water and measure what urine you void from the bladder and then, using ultrasound equipment, measure what is retained. The idea was to void more than one retains. At the start I was going every ten minutes, voiding 200ml but retaining 200+ml. After about five goes I slowed down to every half hour and started voiding 150ml and retaining 40 to 50ml. During this time, I had a visit from the registrar, who said if the void/retain balance kept at the lower retain ratio I could go home. Note the surgical nurse's experience was to do three tests and that was it, so the urology experience was new to them. Nurse Debbie was very good, explaining things and found us plenty of sample pads and knickers.

Recovery Period

So here I am, back in nappies. Life goes full circle. Though did not think I would get the sensation of a full bladder for a while and just dribble. The bladder is giving warning signs – but the dribbling is alive and well during any sharp movement e.g. getting in out of a car, sitting on a seat. It is now time to get pelvic exercises going.

It's all up to me!

Monday, 30th November: overnight got up four times based on a need to empty my bladder. Made it to the toilet every time, only slight dribbles. Some flows quite strong.

Walked over two kilometres with Sue to get paper – no leakage. After breakfast, swept up yard and swept the pool – no leakage. Experienced more leakage around sitting down and standing up.

Over the next four days, keeping up exercises and starting to walk in the afternoon some six-plus kilometers.

Finding that my voiding during the day is stress-related – non-based on a controlled message. In the evening it appears urge-based and I am passing a reasonable flow, but still four to six times per night. Is this the leftover from my previous brain reaction when bladder was blocked by the enlarged prostate?

I am in myself feeling okay but frustrated with lack of control still but it is only the fourth day after my catheter removal. Today, back in the car and picked up Peter Dornan's book *Conquering Incontinence*.

I am following Peter's regime in the book and hope I start to see some improvement over next few weeks. I must be patient as could take months!

I am trying to follow a normal routine and ignoring my body's actions – when it comes down to it, it is all about ridding the body of cancer.

It is now Sunday, 6th December, nineteen days to Christmas. I am still a four-pad-per-day and one-per night person. I seem to be under control at night but completely out of control during the day – that's with using pelvic muscles as much as possible, though this does seem to push the void out, not hold it back. I am trying to ignore my leakage and carry on life as usual; I am managing to walk a least 6–8 kilometres per day in two sessions. A quote from the Dalai Lama: 'If you are able to transform adverse situations into factors of the spiritual path, hindrances will become favourable conditions for spiritual practice.'

This week becoming more active and, on Thursday, started back in the gym. On Wednesday visited the prostate support meeting and picked up some good tips on diet. We also had a singsong for Christmas.

Christmas fun over now into Boxing Day Test and Sydney to Hobart yacht race. Managed to get a two-and-a-half-hour walk in at Mt Cootha on Boxing Day and went well. Of the seven walkers, four were minus their prostate. So this week kept up gym and pelvic exercises – the number of voids at night dropping but still unable to get the voiding message during the day. Standing up the worst time and am trying to pull muscles up at this time with little effect at present. The incontinence frustrating and especially when you hear of others having no issues after two weeks.

It's now a week later and have since had my visit with Dr X. He confirmed the operation went well, though the histological information noted a focal positivity in regards to marginal status. Another new set of indicators, which could indicate the spreading of the cancer – again there is some uncertainty regarding how good the test is and what it means. Dr X was of the opinion that it was maybe caused by the operation. So it is still a waiting period, as PSA will give us the ultimate result. Dr X did give me the opportunity to do a PSA now, but indicated it is better to give it some time so we have decided to wait until the end of January when Dr X returns from holiday. The good news this week is incontinence seems to be on the mend in the last two days and there has been a great improvement and the message seems to be getting through – from brain to bladder.

Continuing with pelvic exercises and building up fitness in the gym and walking. (Will try to get a longer walk in soon, up to five hours.) I guess my only nagging doubt is the focal positivity report but remain positive and am sure the PSA will come up trumps.

It is now the 24th January and life is on the improve, incontinence is nearly under control – since my last report have done a hard twenty-five-kilometre walk of 6.5 hours (a fair bit of leakage); also visited Sydney, meeting friends, both personal and work. Gained a lot more confidence and was able to do all the things I would normally do and certainly feeling fit. Met an old friend from Cape Cabarita days who has been diagnosed with prostate cancer – PSA 16 (last year his PSA was low), regretfully unable to operate as in lymph glands, and is now on hormone treatment. This cannot be a cure, just a control; 'what a bastard this thing is'. Derek seemed to be coping very well but the uncertainty about the future must be tough. (He has since died.) The coming week will be interesting as I will be having my first PSA test since the operation.

Friday, 29th January – 'great news' after giving blood yesterday for my first PSA test. THE RESULT: Point 01. This is an indication that I am clear of cancer. So the first part of the journey is over; the issues of incontinence and erectile dysfunction will take time and are subject to the body repairing itself and fitness. PSA checks will continue over the next couple of years but yesterday's result is a good, positive start. In two weeks off to New Zealand – hooray! – and planning in October my pilgrimage on the Camino de Santiago, a 750-kilometre walk in Spain.

After my holiday in NZ, I have succeeded in ridding myself of pads and my bladder is working well, though no sign of an erection and realise that will take time.

I finish my narrative with a quote from the Dalai Lama:

'I believe each human being has the potential to change, to transform one's own attitude, no matter how difficult the situation. We are human beings, and we have this marvelous brain and marvelous heart, so there is potential to develop a proper mental attitude through which we can have a happy, more peaceful life.'

Don't Put It Off

Warren Cox

It began when I found I could no longer wee,
especially during the night.
It came out in spits and sometimes in spurts,
and I thought to myself, *Hell, That doesn't seem right!*
When I thought I was finished, I wasn't, you see,
'cos *drip, drip... drip, drip* kept bothering me.
So I said to the missus, 'My plumbing's affected.'
She said, 'Darl' It's probably badly connected.
You know, when you start to get long in the tooth
there are signs to remind you you're not bullet-proof.
So I think that it's time an appointment we make.
Off to the doctor, before it's too late.'

So she did. And when first up Doc put on a glove
I stepped back a pace and said, 'Hang about, love!
I hope you're not thinkin' what I think you're thinkin'.'
But she was. And she did. And I tell ya fair dinkum,
the end of the bedrail I firmly took hold.
I nipped and I tucked. And I squirmed and I rolled,
then at last it was over I sat up and waited
while she told me my prostate was large and quite dated.

'It's not a big problem, you'll need a rebore.
Take the stress off your bladder. It won't even be sore.
The bit we remove we'll send off to be checked.
Make sure it's healthy to keep you on deck.'
But the Doc phoned next week and here comes the crunch.
The news that she gave really put me off my lunch.
'The pathology's back and you won't like the answer.
I'm sorry to say that your prostate has cancer.
There are several treatments you've heard of, no doubt,
and though I believe we should just take it out,
the final decision is still yours to make.
You should know what's in store if your prostate I take.'

So I asked her to tell me what problems I'd face
if the prostate was finally removed from its place.
She told me that guys often raised an objection
when told that they'd no longer get an erection.
Then my wife interrupted with this sage remark,
'He's an old dog. His bite is much less than his bark.
It's been ages since he carried on like a pup.
These days, he needs splints to keep it all up.
So if leaving it in still raises a doubt,
I agree with you, Doc, just take it all out.'

A number of thoughts then rolled 'round my head,
but finally I simply chose not to be dead.
Now my PSA rating has dropped below one
and I'm glad I decided to get the job done.
So if your pipe's leaky, if your wee is in strife,
See your doc early. It may just save your life.

Glossary

Active surveillance – When the progress of prostate cancer is closely monitored through regular prostate-specific antigen blood tests, digital rectal exams and ultrasounds.

Anaesthesia – Drugs that cause insensibility (locally or generally) to the body, which then allows surgery to be performed.

Anaesthetist – A doctor who specialises in anaesthesia.

Antidepressants – Drugs that are prescribed to treat depression and other mental disorders.

Asymptomatic – Without symptoms.

The Big C – Colloquialism for cancer.

Brachytherapy – A form of radiation treatment where radioactive seeds are placed directly into the organs or tissues affected by the tumour.

Bio resource – A company which collects and distributes cancer samples from patients to medical researchers.

Biopsy – Examination of tissue samples to find out whether that tissue is cancerous.

Cardiologist – A doctor who specialises in the heart.

Casodex – A drug used to block the action of the male hormones in the prostate. This slows the growth of tumours.

Catheter – A thin tube inserted into the body to remove fluid, usually the bladder.

Chemotherapy – The use of anti-cancer drugs to destroy cancer cells.

Codeine – A drug derived from morphine that is used for analgesic purposes.

Computerised Axial Tomography (CAT) scan – An x-ray that produces cross section views of the anatomy.

The Da Vinci robot – A robotic surgical system that enhances a surgeon's vision and dexterity so they can perform an operation with minimal invasion to the patient.

DRE (Digital Rectal Examination) – An inspection of the rectum and surrounding body parts for abnormalities in shapes and textures of the area by the doctor inserting a finger into the rectum. Commonly referred to as 'The Finger Test'.

Electrocardiogram (ECG) – A medical test that detects heart anomalies by measuring the electrical activity of the heart.

Endocrinologist – A doctor who deals predominantly with the endocrine glands.

Enema – An injection of fluid into the bowel through the rectum to clear the bowel or relieve constipation.

External Beam Radiotherapy – A treatment where an external source of radiation is focused into the body.

Fistula – An abnormal or surgically made opening between two organs or an organ and the body's surface.

Focal positivity report – A report which explains the likelihood of a cancer relapse and if any of the cancer may not have been removed.

Gleason score – The score that predicts how fast spreading the cancer is. After a biopsy is done, the tissue is analysed under a microscope and given two ratings: a primary and a secondary, the Gleason score being the total of these numbers. The more uniform the pattern in the tissue, the lower the score and the less aggressive the cancer is likely to be. The more the variation in the tissue, the higher the score and the more aggressive the cancer is.

High Intensity Focused Ultrasound (HIFS) – A procedure using high-intensity focused ultrasound radiation to remove diseased or damaged tissue.

Hormone therapy (also called androgen deprivation therapy) – Aims to reduce the levels of male hormones in the body through injections, oral medications or surgery.

Ileostomy – When the rectum isn't working properly a surgical opening is created in the abdominal wall to remove waste.

Intravenous cannula – A small tube inserted into a vein to give access to the bloodstream.

'Keyhole' robotic procedure – A minimally invasive surgery that uses cameras and long tubes inserted through 5–10-millimetres wide holes.

Laparoscopic radical prostatectomy – A non-invasive procedure to remove all or part of the prostate using 3D imaging and keyhole surgery.

Magnetic Resonance Imaging (MRI) – A scanning procedure that uses a magnetic field to generate signals from the body and processes them into images.

Naturopath – An alternative form of medicine which uses a wide range of natural treatments.

Nerve-sparing surgery – During the removal of the prostate the doctor will try to save the nerves on either side which produce erections.

Neurologist – A doctor who specialises in the nervous system.

Nomogram – A prediction tool that uses statistical data to help cancer patients understand their disease.

Oncologist – A doctor who specialises in treating cancer.

Open surgery – Surgery which involves a long incision being made to allow doctors see the affected area and use instruments through the opening.

Perineum – The area between the scrotum and the anus.

Physiotherapist – A medical professional who works with patients who have difficulty with their movement as a result of physical injury or disease.

Prostatectomy – The surgical removal of the prostate.

PSA (Prostate-Specific Antigen) test – A test that determines how much prostate-specific antigen is resident in the blood, which can indicate the likelihood of cancer of the prostate, but cannot in itself determine whether cancer is present.

Radiotherapy – The use of targeted x-rays to destroy cancer cells.

Serotonin – A chemical created by the human body that is thought to affect sleep, digestion, mood and memory.

Transperineal biopsy – Small samples of the prostate are taken by inserting a needle into the body through the perineum, the area between the scrotum and anus.

Transurethral resection of the prostate (TURP) procedure – A surgical procedure where portions of the prostate gland are removed through the penis.

Urologist – A urinary and genital tract doctor.

Vascular bundles – Neurovascular bundle: a group of nerves, arteries, veins and lymphatics that travel together.

Watchful waiting – A process of allowing time to pass before giving therapy or medicinal intervention. Repeated testing is sometimes involved.

Zoladex – A drug used to treat cancers that overstimulates the production of certain hormones, which causes that hormone production to shut down.

Zytiga – An oral prescription medication prescribed to treat prostate cancer.

References

Throughout Below the Belt, *our contributors have referenced various internet sites or books, which you may like to look into for research and information.*

Andrology Australia
https://www.andrologyaustralia.org/

Australian Urology Associates
http://www.aua.com.au/

Beyond Blue
http://www.beyondblue.org.au/

Bio Resource
http://www.bioresources.com.au/

The Cancer Council Australia
http://www.cancer.org.au/
Also check the web for the Cancer Council in your state.

Conquering Incontinence
Peter Dornan, Allen & Unwin 2003

Eating for Recovery (Ian Gawler CD)
http://www.iangawlerwebstore.com/product/eating-for-recovery

How to Fight Prostate Cancer and Win
Ron Gellatley, 2000 Cargel Press International

Living Now (Free magazine)
http://www.livingnow.com.au/

Localised Prostate Cancer: A Guide for Men and their Families
Available from the Cancer Council

MedicineNet website
http://www.medicinenet.com/

Medscape website
http://www.medscape.com/

Memorial Sloan-Kettering Prostate Cancer
http://www.mskcc.org/cancer-care/adult/prostate

Nova (Free magazine)
http://www.novamagazine.com.au/

Peter MacCallum Cancer Centre
http://www.petermac.org/

Prostate Cancer Foundation of Australia (PCFA)
http://www.prostate.org.au/

Prostate Cancer: Your Guide to the Disease, Treatment,
Options & Outcomes
Prem Rashid
http://www.prostatebook.com.au/

Prostate Health website
http://www.prostatehealth.org.au/

Shine-A -Light group, Sydney
http://www.acon.org.au/mens-health/cancer/shine-a-
light

St Vincent's Prostate Cancer Centre
http://www.prostate.com.au/

Title:
Journey: Experiences with Breast Cancer

Publication Date:
20 February 2012

Format:
Paperback
(150x230mm, 326 pages)

ISBN:
978 0 987 1538 0 7

Category:
Nonfiction

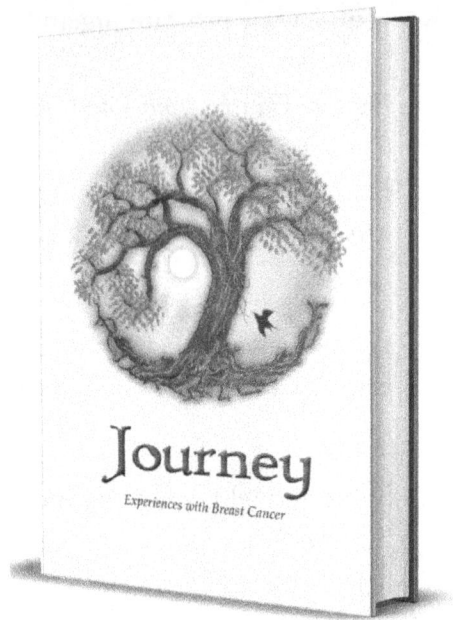

Take a journey with everyday people as they share their experiences with breast cancer. Their stories and poetry are heartfelt and invaluable, offering insights into every facet of their travails: diagnosis, treatment, coping, recovery, and loss. These are people who could be your family, who could be your friends.

There is a strength which comes with sharing. In reaching out and touching others, we build communities of knowledge and assurance. We let each other know that we are not alone.

A portion of proceeds from the sale of *Journey* will go to BreaCan and WHOW (Women Helping Other Women).

Title:
Walk With Me

Publication Date:
22 November 2014

Format:
Hardcover
(300x300mm, 106 pages)

ISBN:
978 0 9925547 2 9

Category:
Coffee Table Book

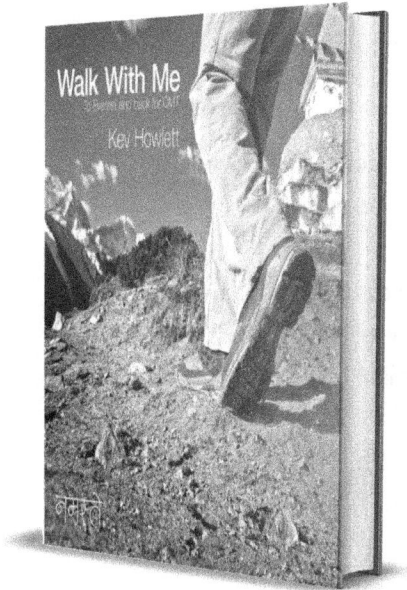

Walk With Me is the trek of Busybird's very own Kev Howlett up to Mount Everest Base Camp and back, detailed in beautiful photography, to raise awareness of Charcot-Marie-Tooth (CMT) disease and funds for the CMT Association Australia.

CMT is an incurable progressive nerve deterioration suffered by 1 in 2,500 people, and a condition also suffered by Kev's own son Dylan. A champion footballer as a teenager, Dylan has had to have both feet reconstructed surgically as a stopgap measure to counter the clawing caused by CMT.

Walk With Me is the journey Kev would've liked to take with Dylan. A photographer with over 25 years experience in the commercial photography industry, Kev details his expedition so that you, too, can walk with him to Everest Base Camp and back and not only enjoy the beauty of Nepal, but also contribute to a good cause.

Title:
The Book Book

Publication Date:
7 February 2014

Format:
Paperback
(181x111mm, 148 pages)

ISBN:
978 0 992 4325 0 8

Category:
Nonfiction

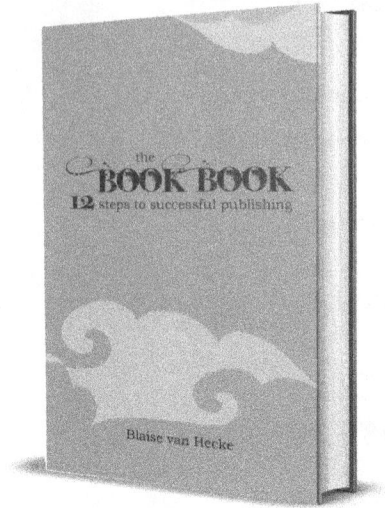

Everyone has a book in them. We all have a story we want to share with the world. But where do we start?

The Book Book will help break the process into small, manageable steps, providing invaluable tips, insider knowledge into the publishing industry, as well as the inspiration to get started and to keep writing to the end.

Don't let this opportunity go to waste!

Trust in *The Book Book* to help you find the way.

Title:
The Launch Book

Publication Date:
22 April 2015

Format:
Paperback
(181x111mm, 70 pages)

ISBN:
978-0-9925226-0-5

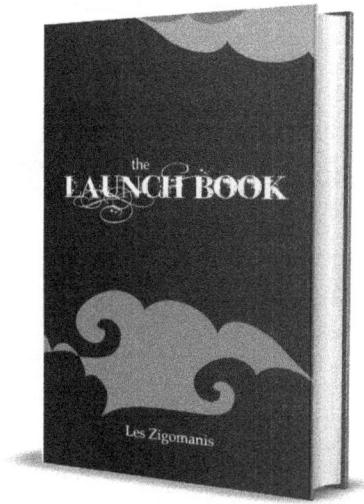

Category:
Nonfiction

You've written and published a book, and you have the first hot copy in your hands.

What's next?

Writing and publishing a book is an incredible achievement, and it shouldn't go unheralded. What a book really needs when it comes into the world is a launch to celebrate its arrival. But what does a launch entail?

The Launch Book is a simple guide that will talk you through the requirements of organising a launch and ensure that all your hard work is duly celebrated.

Title:
The Road to Tralfamadore is Bathed in River Water

Publication Date:
8 August 2018

Format:
Paperback (216x140mm)

ISBN:
Paperback: 978-1-925830-10-1
Ebook: 978-1-925830-03-3

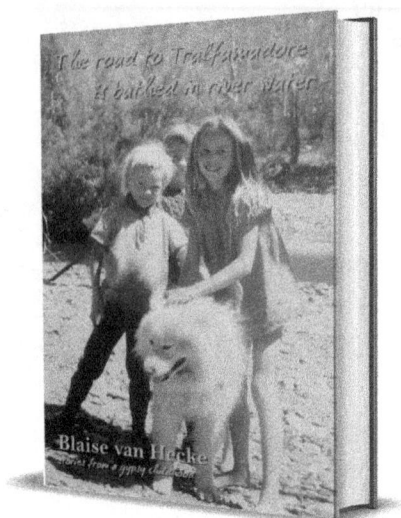

Category:
Nonfiction

In the early 1970s, a single mother and her four children find themselves alone on the east coast of New South Wales. They join the 'Back to the Earth Movement' at the idyllic land known as 'Tralfamadore'.

Lyn and her children choose a spot on a hill bound by a river and creek, building a home using river stones and found objects. They sustain themselves on homegrown produce and fresh air. For Blaise and her siblings, life is unrestrained and full of adventure.

The Road to Tralfamadore is Bathed in River Water is a memoir that depicts a childhood full of both naivety and wisdom during an era of radical social change.

> 'This book captures the innocence and spontaneity of a
> child's view of the world, tempered by the child's wry, sharp,
> affectionate observations on the antics of the wayward, loving,
> flawed, yet wise adults that weave in and out of her life.'
> – Arnold Zable
> Writer, novelist and storyteller.

Title:
50 Days for Fifty Years

Publication Date:
22 January 2020

Format:
Paperback
(178x126mm, 228 pages)

ISBN:
978-1-925949-60-5

Category:
Memoir

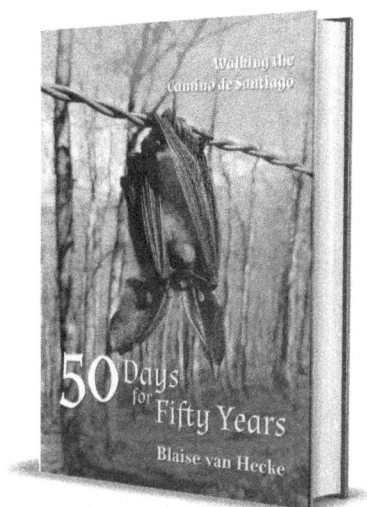

Blaise sets off to celebrate her 50th birthday to give gratitude for her life – a walk of 50 days for fifty years, following the Way of St James in the north of Spain.

What Blaise learns on the Camino de Santiago is gradual, just like the step-by-step journey of over 800 kilometres by foot.

With each passing day, the pilgrimage brings more knowledge and understanding into her heart. Beliefs she's always carried buried blossom into truths that remain with her well after she returns home to Australia.

50 Days for Fifty Years is a gorgeous full-colour memoir that celebrates our journey through life, and the realisations we come to on a long, contemplative sabbatical.

Title:
Pride

Publication Date:
27 April 2017

Format:
Paperback (white cover)
Hardback (red cover)
(234x156mm, 292 pages)

ISBN:
Print: 978-1-925585-24-7
Hardback: 978-1-925585-89-6
Ebook: 978-1-925585-25-4

Category:
Fiction

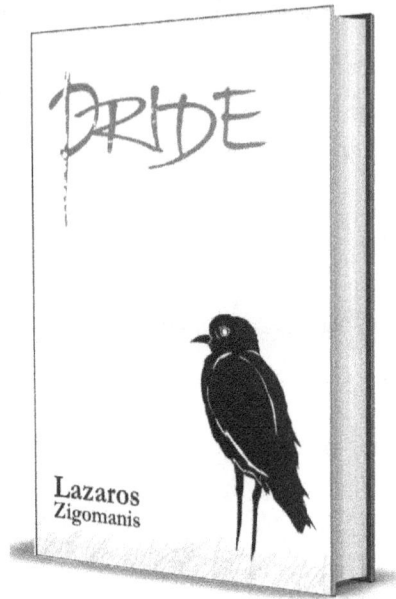

Luke Miggs wants more than what small-town life can offer – the grind of chores on the family farm, playing footy, and drinks with friends. Like maybe doing something about his crush on Amanda Hunt, a barmaid at the local who's smart, funny, and ambitious. Or playing footy in the big league. At 18, it can't be too late, can it?

There are the Ravens, at least, although the team's little more than battlers. If only they could take their footy seriously, like the reigning champions, the Little Reach Scorpions. Under their tyrannical coach, Claude Rankin, the Scorpions have dominated the competition for ten years. It seems nothing will be different this season.

But when Adam Pride emerges from the night and tells the Ravens he wants to play for them, everything begins to change.

Pride is a story of friendship and bonds and coming of age, and how the choices of our past can come back to shape our future.

Title:
The Colours of Ash

Publication Date:
15 May 2022

Format:
Paperback (white cover)
Hardback (red cover)
(234x156mm, 292 pages)

ISBN:
Print: 978-1-925585-24-7
Hardback: 978-1-925585-89-6
Ebook: 978-1-925585-25-4

Category:
Fiction

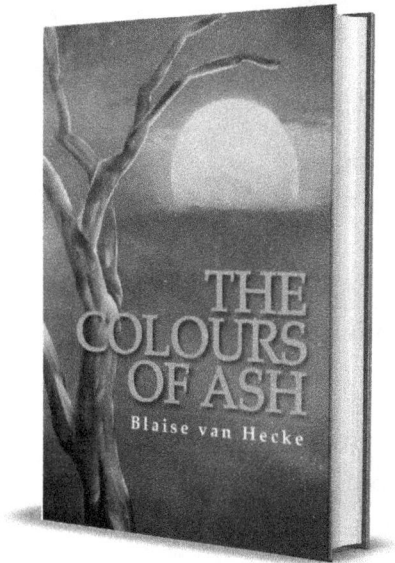

Ash and Destiny enjoy a happy fe in Melbourne with their young son, Tomas, a large and slightly dysfunctional family, a successful art gallery, and Destiny's new exhibition about to debut. But everything changes for Ash on one extremely hot Summer Solstice when a car crash leaves his family shattered.

Waking in hospital Ash knows his whole life has been flipped on its head and his long journey to adjusting to loss and pain is just about to begin. But as time passes both Ash and Destiny struggle to return to their normal life in Melbourne.

When all seems to be lost and stagnating in their lives, the option to move to country Victoria presents itself. An unlikely move for the city-dwelling couple turns into a new and rejuvenating experience that is the start of a new family, but what else does life hold in store?

'A touching and beautiful novel of life, love and family.'
 – Ryan O'Neill
 Their Brilliant Careers 2017 Prime Minister's Literary Award for Fiction

'A shimmering portrait of grief and love, art and life.'
 – Kim Lock
 The Other Side of Beautiful

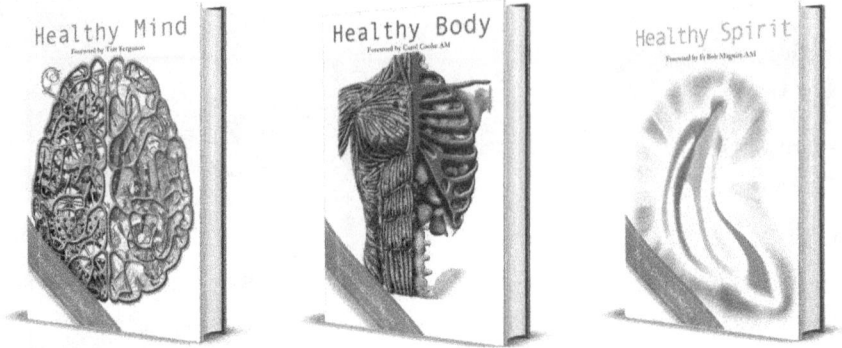

Title:
The Health Conscious Project Series

Format:
Softcover (210x135mm)

Category:
Nonfiction

The Health Conscious Project Series explores a different aspect of health in each of it's books – from the obvious physical and psychological standpoints, to an exploration of cultural and environmental contributors and their impact on our everyday lives.

Healthy Minds is the first book – an anthology that contains articles from diverse professionals, each using their specific expertise to offer tips and exercises on creating and maintaining good mental health.

Healthy Body features articles from various professionals who explore the concept of a healthy body from their specific viewpoint, and offer tips and exercises on creating and maintaining good physical health.

Healthy Spirit is the third instalment, featuring insightful articles from regular people. The articles are written to be interesting and useful to you in their differing ideas about what spirit is and how to care for it.

www.ingramcontent.com/pod-product-compliance
Lightning Source LLC
Chambersburg PA
CBHW020253030426
42336CB00010B/737